The Neck Pain Handbook

*Your Guide to Understanding
and Treating Neck Pain*

The Neck Pain Handbook

*Your Guide to Understanding
and Treating Neck Pain*

GRANT COOPER, M.D.
Princeton Spine and Joint Center
Princeton, New Jersey

ALEX VISCO, M.D.
East Coast Spine, Joint, and Sports Medicine
Hoboken, New Jersey

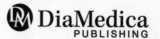 DiaMedica
PUBLISHING

DiaMedica Publishing, 150 East 61st Street, New York, NY 10065
Visit our website at *www.diamedicapub.com*

Library of Congress Cataloging-in-Publication Data
Cooper, Grant, M.D.
  The neck pain handbook : your guide to understanding and treating neck pain / Grant Cooper, Alex Visco.
     p. cm.
  Includes index.
  ISBN 978-0-9793564-8-3 (alk. paper)
1. Neck pain—Handbooks, manuals, etc.   2. Neck pain—Treatment—Handbooks, manuals, etc.   I. Visco, Alex, 1970–   II. Title.
  RC936.C67 2009
  617.5'3—dc22
                                                            2009010560

ISBN: 978-0-9793564-8-3

Note to Readers
This book is not a substitute for medical advice and assistance. The judgment of individual physicians and other medical specialists who know you and who manage the treatment of any medical issues you may have is essential.

Editor: Jessica Bryan
Designed and typeset by: TypeWriting

Printed in Canada

*To my wife Ana, my heart and soul, my partner through everything.
Without her, none of this would be possible.
And to Mila, the newest addition to our family (GC).*

To Shawn, Alexandra, and Vivian (AV).

Contents

Preface   ix

Acknowledgments   xi

About the Authors   xiii

I   Getting to Know Your Neck   1

1   Neck Pain: A New Epidemic   3

2   Learn to Appreciate Your Neck   13

3   When Good Necks Go Bad   23

II   Taking Care of Your Neck   29

4   Posture and the Neck-Friendly Workplace   31

5   Do It Yourself: Simple and Effective
     Exercises for Your Neck   45

6   When Home Exercise Isn't Enough:
     Time to See the Doctor!   59

7   Prescriptions for Conservative Care   71

III Medical Solutions   77

8   Advanced Imaging Studies and
     Trigger Point Injections   79

9   Medications for Neck Pain   87

10   X-Ray-Guided Injections and Surgery   93

IV   Alternative and Complementary Solutions   103

11   Supplements   105

12   Acupuncture and Manual Manipulation   113

13   Meditation   119

14   Concluding Thoughts—Putting It All Together   123

Index   125

Preface

As physicians who specialize in spine and musculoskeletal medicine, we see a steadily increasing number of patients with neck pain. For some, the pain is an occasional nuisance. For many others, it is chronic and severe, interfering with most aspects of their day.

Neck pain doesn't just hurt. It's distracting. It makes it difficult to concentrate on important tasks at home and work. The pain makes it hard to go to the gym or play with your kids; it's fatiguing, and generally makes life difficult. But we have some good news for neck pain sufferers. By taking a few pro-active steps, including reading this book, you can start to substantially reduce your pain *today*.

We will discuss everything you need to know about neck pain, including its causes, how you may be able to treat it yourself, when it's time to see a doctor, and what your doctor can do to help you. Most importantly, we'll discuss how you can *prevent* neck pain, so that once your pain is gone, it will stay gone.

A major contributor to neck pain—and the most important single reason for its steady increase—is the fact that our work situations are increasingly sedentary. We work long hours, and use our computers and e-mail rather than walking down the hall to meet with colleagues, for example. And, we often do this with little attention to posture, hunching over our computer or holding our phones in awkward positions. Immobility for hours on end combined with poor positioning of the neck and shoulders ultimately leads to severe pain. Does this sound like you?

Whatever the cause of your neck pain, the key to choosing the right treatment includes a consideration of the risks and benefits of potential therapies. We emphasize a conservative approach to therapy if there is no evidence of serious injury or other causes of the pain, most often starting with physical therapy. We also recommend the careful and limited use of pain medications initially, to avoid their side effects, adding them into the treatment plan as needed.

Chapters focus on:

- ▶ the importance of good posture while sitting, standing, walking, and sleeping;
- ▶ setting up your workplace for optimal comfort and support, to prevent injury;
- ▶ a simple and effective 10-minute exercise program for your neck, including stretches and strength training, that will help to take away the pain and keep it from coming back;
- ▶ medical options when improving posture and simple exercises don't help;
- ▶ a discussion of the symptoms that mean a physician should be consulted;
- ▶ the approaches that will be used if medical intervention is needed; and
- ▶ options such as medications, injections, and—rarely needed—surgery, for the 10–20% of people with neck pain that does not respond to conservative therapy.

We hope that you will find this book a helpful guide to managing your neck pain, hopefully eliminating it permanently, with safe, effective approaches that will lead to an improvement in your overall health and wellness.

Grant Cooper, M.D.
Alex Visco, M.D.

Acknowledgments

Thank you to Alex's wife, Shawn for posing as the perfect model, and to Todd Kiduff for giving us a great "Ted" model. Thank you to Chris Amaral for his wonderful photography in the book. As always, thanks are due to Dr. Diana M. Schneider and DiaMedica Publishing. Diana is a terrific editor and publisher and we feel lucky to have her collaboration on this and our other projects together.

About the Authors

GRANT COOPER, M.D. is a physical medicine and rehabilitation physician who specializes in the nonoperative treatment of spine, joint, muscle, and nerve pain. He is the co-director of the Princeton Spine and Joint Center in Princeton, New Jersey.

Dr. Cooper has received national and international recognition for his research and publications, and is currently co-editor-in-chief of *Current Reviews in Musculoskeletal Medicine*. His most recent publication is *The Arthritis Handbook* (DiaMedica, 2008). He has appeared on ESPN Radio, National Public Radio, and previously hosted "Back Pain Radio" on World Talk Radio. Dr. Cooper is a consultant to Health Central's Osteoarthritis Center and is on the Medical Advisory Board of the CAN DO Fitness Center.

ALEX VISCO, M.D. is a physical medicine and rehabilitation specialist, a staff physician at Hoboken University Medical Center in Hoboken, New Jersey, and the founder and medical director of East Coast Spine, Joint & Sports Medicine in Hoboken. He specializes in the care of painful conditions of the spine, joints, and muscles, including sports-related injuries. His practice promotes a multidisciplinary approach to patient care and places special emphasis on functional improvement without surgery.

Dr. Visco frequently lectures on the causes and treatment of neck and back pain.

Part I

Getting to Know Your Neck

Neck Pain: A New Epidemic

"I'm 35 years old, and my neck is killing me!"

Do you work long hours and have neck pain? If so, you're not alone. As physicians who specialize in spine and musculoskeletal medicine, it seems as if every day we see more patients with neck pain. For some, the pain is an occasional nuisance. For many others, it is chronic and severe, interfering with most aspects of their day. After all, neck pain doesn't just hurt. It's distracting. It makes it difficult to concentrate on important tasks at home and work. It makes it hard to go to the gym or play with your kids; it's fatiguing, and in general it just makes life difficult. But we have some good news for neck pain sufferers. By taking a few proactive steps, including reading this book, you can start to substantially reduce your pain *today*.

We will discuss everything you need to know about neck pain, including its causes, how to treat it yourself, when it's time to see a doctor, and what your doctor can do to help you. Most importantly, we'll discuss how you can *prevent* neck pain, so that once your pain is gone, it stays gone.

We'd like to start by telling you the story of one of our patients. We believe that much of his story might sound familiar because it might remind you of *you*. His name is Ted. He is 35 years old and works as a financial analyst for a small mutual fund.

Ted had always been an upbeat guy, in good physical condition, and he had never been to the doctor for anything more serious than a bad cold. He ate a healthy diet, never smoked, worked out at the gym three times a week, and once ran the New York City marathon.

Sounds like a guy in perfect health, right? Well, when he first came to see us, he was miserable. He was suffering every day with agonizing neck pain, and could barely turn his head from side to side without a great deal of discomfort. As he talked to us, Ted kept massaging his upper back and neck, clearly in significant pain. He had trouble telling us when all of this started, but it seemed to be getting worse. He didn't like taking pills but sometimes took Tylenol®, aspirin, or Advil® to take the edge off. Still, the only thing that really made his neck feel any better was when he finally lay down to sleep at night.

Ted's experience is typical of many of our patients. Their pain usually comes on gradually and ultimately interferes with most of their everyday activities. Some patients report that they "slept wrong" and had terrible neck pain when they woke up, and that the pain just got worse during the day and never went away. When we question them more closely, however, they can usually remember their necks hurting at some point in the recent past. Sleeping on it "wrong" was just the trigger that put them over the edge.

As with many of our patients, Ted's pain was hurting more than just his neck. It was affecting every part of his life. He had trouble concentrating at work, and he was unusually irritable with his wife. Lifting and playing with his young daughter was simply no longer an option. Ted had a good life, and he wanted to live it. But the pain kept getting in the way. Even worse, although Ted knew he was in pain, he did not know why.

Ted is not the only person with this kind of story, or this kind of pain. Why *would* a healthy 35-year-old man with no medical problems suffer from so much from neck and upper back pain?

We wanted to get a complete understanding of Ted's day. We asked him to describe his typical workday in detail, from the moment he wakes up to the moment he comes home. Here is what he said:

TED'S DAY

"Each morning, I wake up at 5:45 A.M., shower, shave, and get dressed. I help my wife with the baby. I have a cup of coffee and drive to the train. I park in the commuter lot and wait for the train, which usually comes within 15 minutes. I take it to midtown Manhattan and walk a block to the subway, and then take the subway to my office. From the subway stop to my office is about one block.

"I get to work about 8 A.M., take the elevator to the 3rd floor, and usually start checking e-mail. I usually have 20–30 e-mails waiting for me. This takes about 30 minutes. I check the *Wall Street Journal* online and a few business magazines. By that time, my secretary typically reminds me of the calls I need to make. I pick up the phone and start working on that. I also spend a good deal of time working on the computer to communicate with clients, usually through our group software program. By noon, more e-mails have piled up, and I have to handle them. Often, I have a telephone conference with a client early in the afternoon. This can take an hour or so. Then I have more phone calls and e-mails and internal team meetings over the phone or by video teleconference for the next several hours. I usually finish up around 6 or 7 P.M. and head home."

We calculated that Ted's average day included 13–14 hours of work and/or commuting. We asked him if most of that time was spent sitting.

"Almost all of it," Ted said. He paused and looked up in the air as if replaying his day. "I guess I walk from the subway to work, but that's less than a block. I spend the rest of the day sitting."

We noted that most of Ted's responsibilities seem dependent upon the technology at his fingertips. "Yes," Ted agreed, "I guess you could say I'm more of a professional e-mailer than a financial analyst these days."

So, we now know that Ted spends most of his time at work sitting at his desk. He gets up early, sits on a train, walks about a block to work. Between e-mail, reports to write, telephone calls, videoconferencing, and breaks that include surfing the web for online information, he hardly ever has to get up!

Does Ted's day sound familiar? It did to us. We hear this story on a daily basis. The phrase that really caught our attention from our conversation with Ted was when he described himself as a "professional e-mailer." We see people who were once lawyers, stockbrokers, administrators, administrative assistants, corporate executives, and consultants who now all claim to be professional e-mailers! They come to us with similar complaints: "My neck hurts...my back feels tight...my shoulders ache...I get neck pain and headaches...I have pain running down my arm..." We think there is a link here. Let us explain, beginning at the beginning.

OUR ANCESTORS AND THE BODIES WE INHERITED

We can say with some certainty that Ted's great, great, great...great, great grandfather was an active man. Our ancestors had to run, jump, hunt, hide, seek, and forage to survive. *They were in almost constant motion.* Only the most mobile would have survived those dangerous times in human history. Their bodies were challenged constantly in a Darwinian game of survival of the fittest. These are the bodies we have inherited.

Our bodies are not only *capable* of great motion, they *rely* on it. If we don't move, our bodies quickly break down. An extreme example of this phenomenon is seen every day in the hospital. Have you ever visited people who have been in the hospital for a number of days or even weeks? You probably noticed that they were weak, and they might have lost weight. Perhaps you noticed that they seemed older than before. Much of this deterioration is caused by immobility. In fact, for every day you spend lying in bed, you need to exercise for 2 days to regain the lost muscle mass. Immobility causes more than just muscle loss and weakness. Lying in bed for long periods of time affects your heart, lungs, mind, nerves, joints, and sexual function. Where does this all lead? It leads to pain.

The link between pain and immobility is what might be termed an "equal opportunity" phenomenon in that it can affect anyone from the highest-level athlete to the couch potato. If an elite professional football player was confined to bed for a week, he would need at least a month of training before he would be ready again for competition. If we confined him to bed for a month, his season would most likely be finished. If and when he did return to practice, his muscles and joints might be more painful, his joints might ache, his tendons might become inflamed, and he might never be able to return to his previous level of play. Our bodies are undeniably designed for motion, and lots of it.

> Our bodies are not only capable of great motion, they rely on it. If we don't move, our bodies quickly break down.

TED BRINGS US BACK TO HIS QUESTION

"Okay, Doc," Ted said to us after we told him about his great, great, great…great ancestors. "That's a terrific story. But what does that have to do with *my* neck and *my* life? Don't you have a pill or something for the pain?"

We asked Ted to be patient. We assured him that we were here to help him, but we had some more questions first.

"I had a feeling there would be more questions. What else could you possibly need to know?"

We told Ted that we wanted to know something about his life before his neck pain, and as we talked more with him, we found out that he wasn't always this immobile at work. He *used* to go to meetings. He *used* to visit colleagues to ask them questions and borrow their files. Not any more. He no longer needs to. For the last 2 years, his office has been wired so that he can get all the files he needs with the push of a button.

Text messaging has replaced many face-to-face conversations. Still other conversations are held on the phone, so that both parties can access information on the computer simultaneously. Meetings? Yes, but not live, in-person meetings. Teleconferencing and videoconferences have done away with Ted's need to leave his desk even for a meeting. He either skips lunch completely, or it is only a phone call away. On an ambitious day, Ted might walk a short distance to get a sandwich. But he rarely has time for even that.

"In many ways," Ted told us, "my life has gotten a lot more convenient and efficient. For the last 2 years, I've hardly ever had to get out of my chair at all."

We asked Ted to try and think about how long he has been experiencing his neck pain.

Ted looked at the ground, shook his head back and forth. He focused back on us. "About 2 years."

You might notice, as we did, that Ted's day seems to more closely resemble that of a bed-ridden hospital patient than that of a healthy, active 35-year-old man. And, while a patient will hopefully stay in the hospital for no more than a few days or weeks, Ted does this 5 days a week, with no end in sight. That's 70 hours of immobility each week! Add 2 hours a day for sitting during his commute and 7 hours each night sleeping, we can see that Ted spends *at least 115 hours each week in a state of near immobility!* That's almost 70 percent of his time!

THE DOUBLE WHAMMY

It appears that Ted is a victim of immobility, and that this immobility might have something to do with his neck pain—but why his *neck* and not another body part? The answer to this lies in the position of Ted's body as he sits at his desk all day.

You can see from Ted's picture of himself at work that he looks pretty uncomfortable. He agreed and said, "Yes, I'm hunched over like

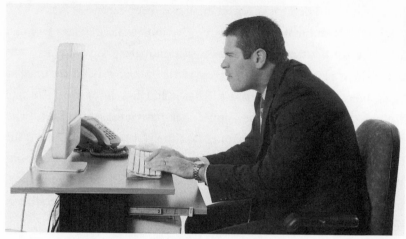

Ted at work. Does this look like you?

that pretty much all day long. I think my body just gets in that position and stays there. I don't have a chance to think about it during the day."

Immobility and Poor Positioning

These are the two aspects of the "Double Whammy," and we see them in our medical practice all day long. This is the heart of Ted's problem, and possibly yours as well. Immobility for hours on end, combined with poor positioning of the neck and shoulders, ultimately leads to severe pain. If Ted does not address these issues soon, the pain might spread to his lower back. People suffering from the Double Whammy typically:

> *Immobility for hours on end, combined with poor positioning of the neck and shoulders, ultimately leads to severe pain.*

- ▶ Work long hours
- ▶ Are relatively immobile for most of the day
- ▶ Spend much of this time in a "hunched over" position at their desk
- ▶ Make significant use of office technology: e-mail, telephone, teleconferencing, computers, and videoconferencing

Although desktop computers have been around for several decades, this problem is getting worse. Technology used to be a tool that we utilized from time to time. Now, it dominates the workplace. It is everywhere. No one makes a move at work without making use of *some* piece of equipment or software. This is hurting all of us, including young, strong people who should *not* have neck and back pain. Computers, e-mail, and telephones take the place of walking down the hall to see colleagues and face-to-face meetings with clients. Slowly but surely, technology has taken away the small but important amount of physical activity we used to take for granted. In Ted's case, he barely moves except to get up to go to the bathroom.

Why did Ted fail to make the connection between his lack of physical activity, his chronic hunched-over position, and his neck pain? It's simple enough, and Ted is a smart guy. But, actually, most of the people we see in our office don't seem to make the connection. We have become so accustomed to technology that we assume that using our computer, e-mailing, and talking on our cell phone are as natural and inevitable as using a toothbrush, eating breakfast, and watching television. We also seem to have accepted the idea that our bodies should adapt to our equipment, instead of the other way around. Perhaps we feel that these things—these tools that make so much possible—can't possibly hurt us.

We need to reassess our physical interaction with the hardware and software in our workplaces, as well as when we work at home.

Wrong!

Our physical interactions with technology are now so automatic that it's hard to recognize the pain they cause us. We need to reassess our physical interaction with the hardware and software in our workplaces, as well as when we work at home.

But we can't throw out the baby with the bathwater!

Let's face facts. E-mail and teleconferences aren't going away anytime soon—nor should they. We still need to compete in the global marketplace.

It *is* possible to use e-mail, text messaging, teleconferences, and videoconferences and remain *pain-free*. We can—in a very real and immediate sense—have it all, and we don't have to invest large amounts of money or make major lifestyle changes to achieve it. We do need to acknowledge the problem, understand what is going on, and then make some straightforward, common-sense adjustments. By taking a few minutes out of your day to do some easy exercises at your desk or during your daily commute, and by making a few simple, inexpensive adjustments to your office equipment, you can reduce and even eliminate your neck pain—and keep it from coming back.

By taking a few minutes out of your day to do some easy exercises at your desk or during your daily commute, and by making a few simple, inexpensive adjustments to your office equipment, you can reduce and even eliminate your neck pain—and keep it from coming back!

After years of seeing patient after patient just like Ted, we know that as soon as we say "daily exercises," a glazed look comes over many people. Who has time for daily exercise? Any doctor who would even suggest such a thing must be disconnected from a sense of reality! Even when we assure our patients that the exercises don't take a significant amount of time, some people still cringe. It's not that our patients with neck and upper back pain fear making the effort. To the contrary, they don't believe they have time to fit *anything* else into their already overly busy lives.

To help them focus on the cause of their pain and possible solutions, we ask them questions such as these:

▶ How much time do you spend during the day thinking about your neck pain?
▶ How much does the pain in your neck distract you and keep you from making your best effort at work?
▶ You know that being pain-free would make your life more enjoyable, but can you also appreciate that it would even make you more productive at everything you do, including work?

▶ If you could truly concentrate at work, do you think it might help you do a better job—maybe even get a promotion?

▶ If you had less pain, would you be more fully engaged with your loved ones?

▶ Would being more engaged with every aspect of your life strengthen your close relationships and improve your overall quality of life?

These questions usually cause resistance to fade, and it is worth taking the time to consider them. Believe us, if there were a magic pill out there to take away your neck pain and keep it from coming back, we'd suggest it. The problem with taking pills for your pain is that they generally only mask the symptoms; they don't address the underlying problem. Also, taking any medication—including those available without a prescription—for a long period of time can have serious health consequences, including stomach and kidney problems. Many of the stronger painkillers also make you sleepy during the day. It is far better and more effective to fix the underlying problem than to mask it with a pill. In Ted's case, as we have seen, the underlying problem is a combination of immobility, body positioning at work, and the way that he uses technology—in fact, it might be fair to say that Ted's technology is using him!

> *The problem with taking pills for your pain is that they generally only mask the symptoms; they don't address the underlying problem.*

As we said, Ted is intelligent. He immediately understood that increasing his ability to concentrate, decreasing the time he spent at work thinking about his neck pain, and improving his overall quality of life was easily worth a small time investment in daily exercises. If making simple, inexpensive adjustments to his technology would help his pain, he was eager to do that as well.

Does Ted's predicament sound similar to your own? Like Ted, are you wondering what exercises you can do at your desk, how to modify your technology, and how to relieve the pain and keep it from coming back?

We can show you how. That's why we wrote this book.

Learn to Appreciate Your Neck

It's easy to take your neck for granted. Most of us do. We expect it to be there for us, day in and day out. We don't expect it to give us any grief. After all, compared to other parts of the body, its job seems downright easy. All your neck has to do is hold up your head while you are awake. And, it gets to rest all night! In contrast, other parts of our body appear to have more vital purposes. The heart pumps tirelessly and constantly regulates blood supply to meet demand. No easy task. The brain coordinates billions of functions every moment of the day and night. The hands and feet are called upon to help us negotiate our environment at a moment's notice. These are all noble purposes, but what about the neck? We take it for granted and don't appreciate how critical it is.

It's time to take another look at the poor, misunderstood neck, because more people than ever before are needlessly suffering from daily, disabling neck pain. We need to appreciate it for what it really is—a biomechanical work of art!

THE NECK IS AN ANATOMIC MARVEL

Typically, most of us think of the neck solely as a support for the head. Imagine the neck in a simple stick figure, like those children often draw. This is a good representation of our oversimplified view of the purpose and function of the neck. Now visualize a giant head held up by one thin vertical line, and then contrast it to the image below, which shows the complexity of the muscles in the neck.

YOUR AMAZING NECK

How many muscles did you think were in the neck before you saw this picture? Most people would guess four, maybe six. In fact, there are more than 20, each of which provides its own unique contribution to the neck's structure, strength, and mobility. These muscles work together to make possible a vast range of movements, including the basic movements of flexion, extension, rotation, and side bending.

Combinations of these movements allow for the virtually unlimited ability of the neck to achieve any desired position. No other part of the body has such a remarkable versatility of movement.

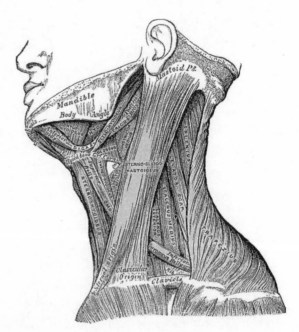

The muscles of the neck.

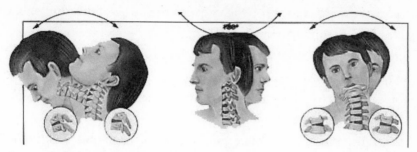

The primary movements of the neck are flexion, extension, rotation, and side bending. With permission of kline18.tripod.com.

Let's look closer at the muscles in the neck. You can see that each has a unique starting and ending point. The point at which a muscle begins is called its point of *origin*, and its ending point is called its *insertion*. The function of an individual muscle depends on its origin and insertion points. For example, two of the largest muscles in the neck are the *sternocleidomastoids* on each side. Their origins are the *sternum* (the breastbone) and the *clavicle* (the collarbone); their inser-

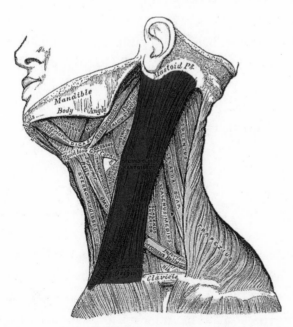

The sternocleidomastoid muscle helps the neck to flex, rotate, and bend to the side.

tion is the *mastoid process*, which is part of the base of the skull on the side of the head. When this muscle contracts, it pulls the points of origin and insertion closer together, which causes the neck to perform a combination movement of flexion, rotation, and bending to the side. You can easily feel this muscle on your own neck. It is the largest muscle on either side.

When you flex and rotate your head at the same time, you can see and feel the sternocleidomastoids contract. This muscle is no different from the biceps muscles in your arms or the quadriceps muscles in your legs in that it contracts to cause a specific movement. The difference is that there are relatively few muscles in the upper arm and leg compared to the neck. When you realize how many muscles there are in the neck—each with its own highly specialized purpose—you can begin to understand its true complexity.

COORDINATING MOVEMENT

With so many muscles pulling and pushing in different directions, you might think that things could get a little chaotic. Certainly there needs to be some adult supervision here?

Certainly there is. Like the conductor of a symphony orchestra, your brain ensures that the many parts of the neck harmonize as one and work together. Each muscle is "hard-wired" through the nervous system to the brain, where the finest of movements are constantly monitored and regulated. If, for example, one muscle is instructed to pull, the brain will simultaneously instruct muscles on the opposite side of the neck to relax. In this way, the brain both causes a movement and prevents resistance to it. Like the conductor who orders the percussion section to soften so the flutist can be heard, the brain maintains discipline in the neck. Think of a seemingly simple movement such as rotating your head back and forth. At the microscopic level, there is nothing simple about it. With so many muscles involved, and so many points of insertion and origin, billions of messages pass through the nerves from the brain to the muscles each second. Not even the most powerful computer in the world can come close to matching this feat!

This orchestra, with the brain as conductor, needs a stage on which to perform a sophisticated symphony of movement. This is where the bones of the neck join the performance. Since the muscles are basically soft, they need a strong support upon which they can push and pull. Here is what your neck looks like without its muscles:

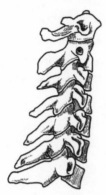

The bones of the cervical spine.

There are seven vertebrae in your neck, stacked on each other to form the *cervical spine*. The spine is the only part of the body where bones are stacked this way, allowing for both the neck's great strength and its remarkable mobility.

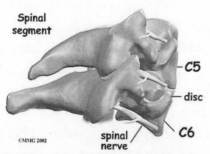

Cervical vertebrae C5 and C6. The facet joints are found where the vertebrae meet behind the discs. eOrthopod (www.eOrthopod.com) image provided as a courtesy of Medical Multimedia Group (www.medicalmultimediagroup.com).

Look at the two vertebrae in the figure above and notice how they are stacked on top of each other. The front part of the bone lies on top of the other, separated by a soft *intervertebral* disc that acts as a kind of shock absorber. We'll talk more about these discs later. The back parts of the vertebrae meet each other at two points called *facet joints*. These are real joints, just like your knees or shoulders. They allow the neck to flex, but they also help limit extension and turning. This means that one vertebra can move in any number of directions with respect to the other, but a mechanical "catching" mechanism is also present that prevents the neck from being *too* flexible. Forward, backward, twisting, and turning movements are all possible to some degree. Now, picture all seven vertebrae stacked together with their shock absorbers and joints held together by flexible ligaments and tendons. You can now begin to appreciate the beauty of segmental design, much like a long freight train.

LIGAMENTS AND TENDONS

Ligaments are tough fibrous bands of tissue that connect bones to other bones, and *tendons* are bands of tissue that connect muscles to bones. Muscles, of course, provide the power for movement.

The next figure shows an overhead view of a cervical spine vertebra.

Notice the hole in the middle of the bone. Each bone of the cervical spine has one. When the bones are stacked upon one another and connected, these holes form the tunnel through which the *spinal cord* travels from the brain to the *coccyx* at the base of the spine. Nerves come off the spinal cord and exit through spaces between the vertebrae. These spaces are called *foramen*.

These nerves then travel to the rest of the body, including the arms, legs, organs, and muscles. This is how the brain communicates with other parts of the body. When you want to raise your arm at the shoulder, for example, a command is sent from the brain, through

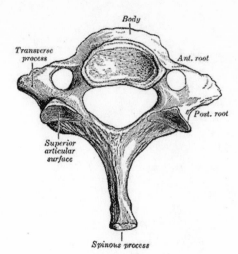

Overhead view of a cervical vertebrae. The spinal cord travels through the large opening in the center.

the spinal cord, and then to a nerve that exits through a space between the vertebrae to the shoulder. If all is well, you will be able to raise your arm.

Spinal cord injuries occur only when a great deal of force is involved; for example, in an automobile accident or a diving injury.

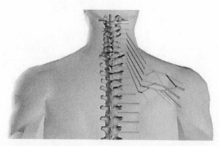

Nerve roots exiting the cervical spine. eOrthopod (www.eOrthopod.com) image provided as a courtesy of Medical Multimedia Group (www.medicalmultimediagroup.com).

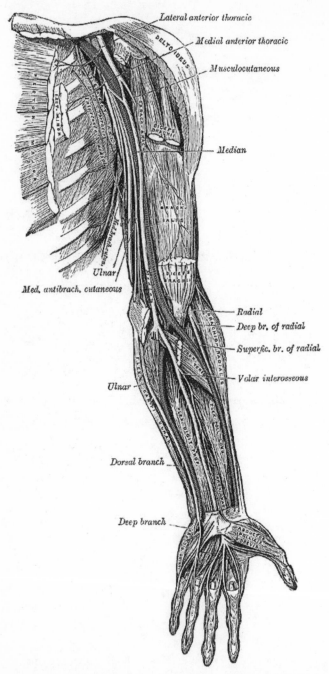

Some cervical nerve roots branch and innervate the muscles and skin of the arms.

TED REFLECTS ON HIS NECK

"I never thought about how important my neck was before. I guess I really have been taking it for granted all these years. You know, I think I'm like most people. I have always been aware of the muscles in my stomach, arms, and legs, but I never thought about taking care of my neck muscles. I guess that's been part of the problem."

We assured Ted that he was, in fact, well within the norm to have not previously considered his neck more thoughtfully. That's why a basic understanding of how your neck works is crucial when it comes time to fix the problem. If you don't appreciate that you're driving a fine automobile, you'll eventually run it into the ground. If you know that you're in possession of a Porsche, you'll make sure that you change the oil on time, feed it top-quality gasoline, rotate the tires, and take it for a spin now and then to let it "flex its muscle." The same is true for your neck. If you appreciate and understand what an incredible machine your neck truly is, you'll understand how to take care of it and—just as importantly—you'll be motivated to actually do so.

Otherwise, these devastating injuries are quite rare. This serves as a testament to the strength of the cervical spine and its supporting structures.

WHY IS MOVEMENT SO NECESSARY?

Why do we need so much movement and strength? Don't we spend most of our time just looking straight ahead? Wouldn't it be better to sacrifice some flexibility for strength and stability?

Remember our great, great, great…great ancestor. Constant vigilance about his environment was vital to survival. If he couldn't quickly turn his head to spot danger, the human race might not have survived. The neck is a biomechanical marvel of evolution, and its capabilities have developed over the millennia to help ensure our survival. Like us, our ancestor collected information through his senses, mostly through hearing and sight. He also had to be constantly alert to the dangers around him, and be able to move fast. Just as the ears and eyes are necessarily located in the head, the neck was key to gathering rapid access to information. Envision your ancestor during flight or fight; head turning, twisting, flexing, and extending to gather crucial life-saving information.

You might think you don't need these same powers, until you find yourself crossing a busy city street during rush hour. Whether you use your neck the same way as your ancestor or not, it helped get you to where you are today—very much alive! The neck is capable of motion because of the way it has evolved, and it *needs* motion.

What do Olympic athletes, thoroughbred horses, and Formula 1 race cars have in common? They are all great performers, and we marvel at their feats and accomplishments. Behind the scenes, they require a good deal of care and attention in order to maintain their highest levels of performance. If they are not attended to, even coddled, they can break down rather easily. The most important structures of the neck evolved as parts of a complex, high-performance biologic machine that requires daily maintenance. Each of its parts can break down in some way or another, resulting in neck pain. With a newfound respect for your neck, and a little care and attention, you can foresee, treat, and avoid many of these problems.

When Good Necks Go Bad

Nerves transmit all sorts of information from the body to the brain, and pain is one of the most important. Without nerves, you couldn't experience pain. For example, the brain itself does *not* have a nerve supply. For this reason, when neurosurgeons perform operations on the brain, they only have to anesthetize the scalp. Once inside the brain, the neurosurgeon can poke and prod with the patient wide awake and feeling no pain.

This makes good evolutionary sense. We experience pain as a danger warning. Your hand on a hot stove sends the message that it is painful, so you'll pull it away. Likewise, a sprained ankle is painful, so that you'll take it easy and allow it to heal. By contrast, the brain—from an evolutionary standpoint—has never needed to express pain as a warning signal because an exposed brain means death.

Many structures in your neck have a nerve supply—and each one can cause pain. The most common sites of pain in the neck are the muscles, tendons, and facet joints.

Muscular Neck Pain

Imagine holding a 10-pound bowling ball over your head for 10 minutes. Now imagine holding that same ball over your head for 18 hours. Well, your head weighs slightly more than that bowling ball, and your neck holds it up all day, every day. If you want your neck to support your head without pain, day in and day out, you need to have optimal body biomechanics and a well-toned neck. The neck muscles are common sources of pain, not only as a result of having to hold up your head all day, but also as a result of an imbalance between the lower neck and chest muscles. Most people tend to pull their shoulders forward, creating a sloped appearance, as you can see in the figure on page 25, because the *pectoral* (chest) muscles are stronger compared to those that pull your shoulder blades backward—the *rhomboids* and *trapezius*. This is in part due to genetics and in part due to our tendency to focus on exercising those muscles we can see in the mirror—the chest, biceps, and front thigh muscles, not what we don't see—the muscles of the upper back, the small stabilizing shoulder muscles, and the buttock muscles.

Optimal posture means having the chin tucked in, the shoulders back, and the head above the neck—not flexed forward, as you can see in the figure on the next page. Without optimal posture, the resulting muscular imbalance leads to a constant strain on the upper back and neck muscles as they try to compensate. This in turn leads to fatigue and spasm and, ultimately, to pain in these muscles.

When you sit at a computer with a screen that is not positioned correctly, you might flex your neck forward even more than usual, as shown on page 26. This is like holding that bowling ball in front of you instead of over your head—it's a much harder task. By positioning the screen so that you look directly at it without flexing your head, and by placing the keyboard closer to your chest, you can avoid hyperflexing your neck and thus spare your muscles from stress (the second picture on page 26).

We'll discuss how to maintain appropriate posture in a variety of common situations in Chapter 4.

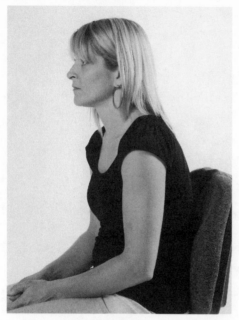

Poor sitting posture with "sloping" shoulders.

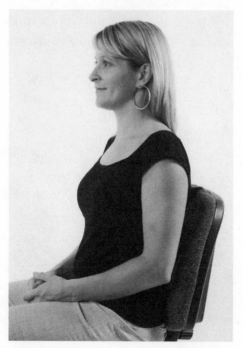

Optimal sitting posture.

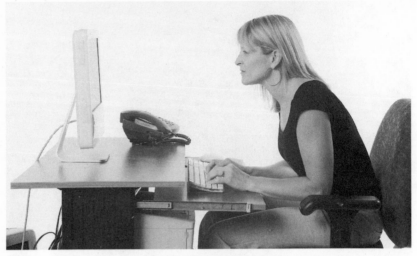

Poor workstation setup. Note that her neck is hyperflexed.

TENDON AND LIGAMENT PAIN

We have seen that neck and upper back muscles are fatigued not only by holding the head up, but also from trying—in a mostly losing battle—to

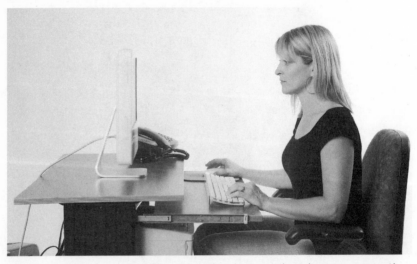

Improved workstation setup. The keyboard and monitor have been repositioned allowing her to have much better posture.

hold our shoulder blades back. This places constant strain on the muscles, which, in turn, leads to tension, soreness, spasm, and pain.

But muscles aren't the only potential source of pain. Muscles are attached to the bones by tendons. These tendons can also become inflamed from the constant tension placed on them. You might think of this as "tendonitis of the neck."

Ligaments attach bones to other bones. The most common ligament to be injured is an ankle ligament, due to a sprain. Although much less common, ligaments in the neck can also be sprained. Again, this occurs most commonly as the result of the constant tension of holding your neck in a suboptimal anatomic position. Ligaments are static structures that have only a certain amount of give and tautness. They can become irritated and painful when they are constantly stretched in a suboptimal position.

Injury to the facet joints is the number one cause of chronic neck pain.

FACET JOINT PAIN

The facet joints are small joints in the back of the spine that allow forward flexion and limit extension and rotation of the spine. Injury to these joints is the number one cause of chronic neck pain. The most common way these joints become injured is in a *whiplash injury*, such as from a motor vehicle accident. However, just like almost any joint in the body—such as the knee, hip, shoulder, or ankle—arthritis can develop in the facet joints as the result of normal wear and tear. When they become arthritic, they can become painful.

The joints in the neck are placed under constant chronic strain when the neck muscles are weak and/or tight, and when body biomechanics are suboptimal. This repetitive strain can result in a wearing down of the joint, which, in turn, can lead to inflammation and pain. When these joints become inflamed and painful, the overlying muscles sometimes spasm in a futile and belated effort to "protect" the joints.

Unfortunately, these muscle spasms only serve to worsen the pain because the spasms themselves are painful, and because they move the joints into suboptimal patterns, further irritating them.

Part II

Taking Care of Your Neck

4

Posture and the Neck-Friendly Workplace

By now you are starting to get the picture that good posture is essential both to treating and preventing neck pain. This means good posture when you walk, when you sit at your desk or in front of the television, drive your car, and even when you sleep. Good posture distributes weight onto structures that are designed to support that weight, and off of structures not designed to support it. Good posture also places your muscles in biomechanically advantageous positions. Bad posture most typically results in a hyper-flexed neck, as you can see on the next page. This places constant strain on the muscles in your neck and upper back.

Good posture is essential both to treating and preventing neck pain.

TED TRIES FOR A QUICK FIX

Ted asked us, "Are you telling me that all I have to do is sit up straight?" and we answered, "Well, not exactly, Ted. But it's not a bad start."

Good posture must be maintained throughout the day. Let's start by reviewing good standing posture.

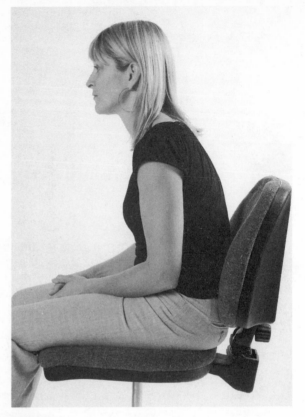

Poor sitting posture.

Good Standing Posture

Stand with your feet shoulder-width apart, as shown on the next page. Don't lock your knees, but bend them slightly. Your weight should be on the balls of your feet—not your heels or toes. Tighten your abdominal and buttock muscles, bringing your pelvis underneath your lower back. Your head should be right on top of your spine, not flexed forward. Stand up straight, with your shoulders falling naturally down and a little back, and your chest out. A good way to check your standing posture is to stand with your heels touching a wall. In this position, the back of your head should touch the wall, as in the figure on the next page.

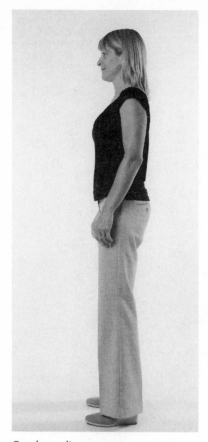

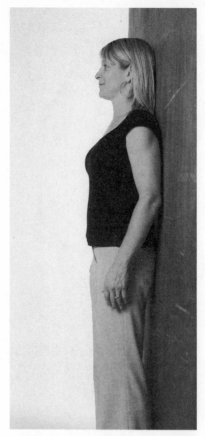

Good standing posture.

Check your standing posture against a wall. Your heels and the back of your head should touch the wall.

The next picture of Ted shows his sloping shoulders and forward-flexed neck. These postural mistakes are very common. He looks a lot more comfortable after correcting his posture.

GOOD WALKING POSTURE

Let's examine good walking posture. Start with good standing posture and, as you walk forward, keep your head squarely above your spine—there is a tendency for the head to lean forward and lead the rest of the

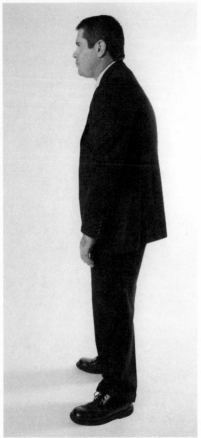

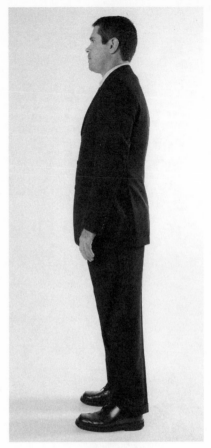

Ted's poor standing posture. His shoulders are sloped forward and his neck is flexed.

Ted's corrected standing posture.

body. Keep your head up and your eyes looking straight out in front of you, as shown on the next page. Of course, if you are walking somewhere such as through a construction site or on a sidewalk with poor paving, you will need to look down a little for safety. Once you have your bearings, remember to put your head back up and try to maintain good posture.

Sometimes, even after mastering good standing posture, you might forget what you've learned when you start walking. Pay attention to your abdominal muscles as you walk. They should contract, to keep

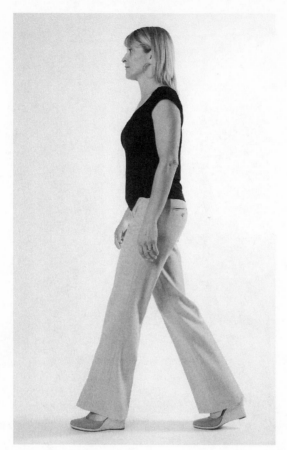

Good walking posture.

you upright and stable. Take a look at Ted's walking posture on the next page. Can you pick out the problems? He is making several common mistakes, including letting his shoulders and neck slouch forward, which we helped him correct.

GOOD SITTING POSTURE

Good sitting posture starts with a good-quality office chair. Ideally, it should be adjustable and *ergonomically* designed to properly support the lower back. (The term "ergonomic" refers to equipment, such as

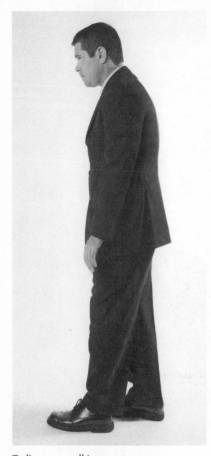 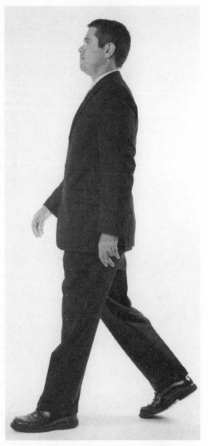

Ted's poor walking posture.

Ted's corrected walking posture. See that his head is now up and looking forward.

chairs and keyboards, designed for optimal positioning and minimal stress on the body, thus preventing repetitive strain injuries and chronic pain.) This doesn't mean it has to be expensive. Your chair should be adjustable, so that you can put the back of the chair at about 90 degrees, and there should be a curve in the back of the chair to provide support for your lower back. However, the best support in the world won't help unless you sit with your back against the chair. All too often, people buy expensive, wonderfully designed chairs, and then sit at the edge of them without taking advantage of the lumbar support. So remember to sit with your buttocks and back against the back of the chair.

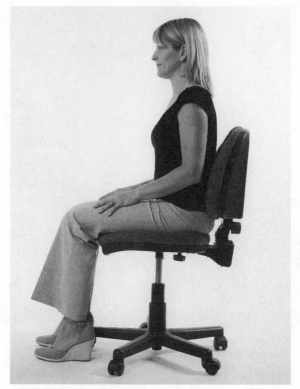

Good sitting posture in an ergonomic office chair.

Your elbows should be flexed at 80–90 degrees.

Your knees should be slightly higher than your hips, such that your fingers can easily slide under your thighs—not too tight a squeeze, but not too much room either. Your feet must be flat on the floor, as shown in the above figure. If the chair is too high and not adjustable, consider putting a foot stool or several phone books on the floor, so that your feet are flat.

Remember that no matter how perfect your posture, you need to change position from time to time. Don't sit in one place for too long. Stand up and stretch often. We'll discuss how to work exercise into your day in Chapter 5.

A number of mistakes are commonly made with seating posture. Look at Ted in his chair, before we helped him. His feet are not on the

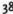

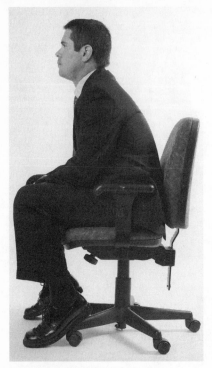 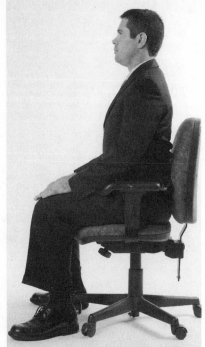

Ted's poor sitting posture.   Ted's corrected sitting posture.

floor, and he is slouching. His neck is flexed forward. This is the posture of someone who is experiencing pain, or who is going to develop pain in the future. He felt much more comfortable after we helped him adjust his sitting posture.

SETTING UP YOUR WORKSTATION

It's time to address your desk or workstation. Remember that you should not need to twist, turn, or bend over in order to accommodate your workstation. Adjust your work environment to accommodate you!

Begin by sitting comfortably and correctly in your chair. Move it as close as is comfortable to your desk. Keep your elbows at an 80–90-degree angle. If your desk is too high or too low, adjust your chair accordingly.

As we mentioned, keep your buttocks against the back of the chair. Its natural contour should provide some lower back (lumbar) support. If it doesn't, place a small cushion behind your lower back. The idea is to have your buttocks against the back of the chair, sitting up straight, with support along your lower back, filling in the natural curve of your spine.

Your chair should have armrests, and you should use them. Set the armrests so that your elbows remain at 80–90 degrees and rest your forearms on the pads. Your shoulders should fall comfortably or be raised slightly from the armrests. This takes some of the strain off your neck, upper back, and shoulders.

Your eyes should naturally look straight ahead, at the center of your computer screen. You should not have to bend forward to look down at the screen. If you do, adjust your screen as shown earlier. Moving the computer screen closer to your eyes will also make it *uncomfortable* to move your head forward, and this will keep you upright as well.

If you spend more than 5 minutes at a time on the phone, or if you spend more than an hour a day (total) on the phone, make sure you have a headset—and are using it. It's time to get rid of your handheld phone.

Here are two pictures of Ted at his workstation. Our necks hurt from just looking at them.

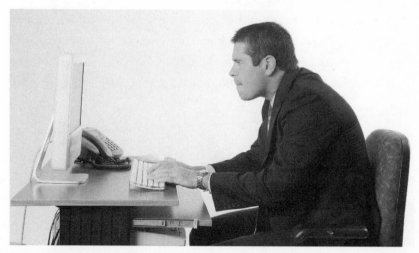

Ted at his desk. His monitor is too low and the keyboard is too far away.

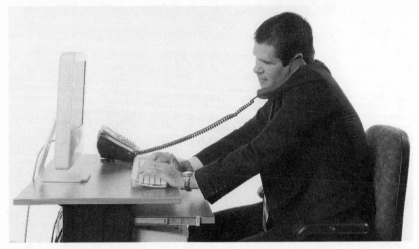

Ted at his desk and on the phone. A headset would be helpful here.

In the first picture, his computer screen is too low and too far away. His keyboard is also too far away, forcing him to reach out to type. This movement places constant strain on the back of Ted's shoulders and on his neck.

In the second picture, see how his neck is crimped to the side as he talks on the phone while working on the computer.

The figures on the next page show Ted after we helped him adjust his posture and workstation. Looking at these pictures makes us feel more relaxed and at ease. His neck no longer strains forward. His chest is opened up instead of pulling his shoulders forward. Ted looks more confident, poised, and comfortable, and he probably feels that way, too.

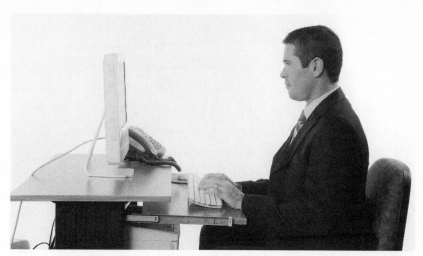

Ted at his desk after our intervention. The monitor and keyboard have been repositioned to help him improve his sitting posture.

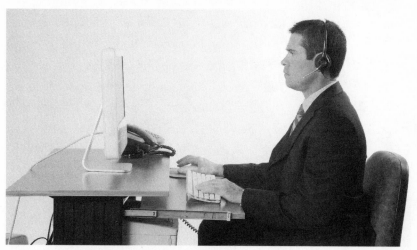

A simple telephone headset can help reduce the risk of neck pain at work.

TED'S PROGRESS

After we showed Ted how to adjust his posture and workstation, he immediately reported feeling a significant improvement. He still had pain, but it was much less. He didn't feel as tired during and after work, and the severe pain he used to have at the end of the day was gone. He achieved all this just from a few simple adjustments.

THE KEY TO HOLDING GOOD POSTURE

Good posture is much easier to maintain when your muscles are well toned and relaxed. A few simple exercises can go a long way toward reducing your pain by improving posture. When your muscles are relaxed and strong, your body will more *naturally* assume the correct anatomic position. The goal in obtaining good body posture throughout your day is to make it *automatic.* For the first few days or weeks, you will have to consciously remind yourself to sit, stand, and walk with good posture. With time, it will become automatic. After a few weeks, you might occasionally fall into your old bad habits, but they will be easy for you to feel, recognize, and correct.

Good posture is much easier to maintain when your muscles are well toned and relaxed. A few simple exercises can go a long way toward reducing your pain by improving posture.

The next chapter offers a set of simple but vital exercises that will keep your muscles loose and strong. You can do them at home or even during the day while at work.

KEEP GOOD POSTURE EVEN WHILE SLEEPING

The best thing you can do for your neck while sleeping is to have a proper mattress and pillow for support. There really is no "best mattress" or "best pillow." There is only a "best mattress and pillow" *for you*. Everyone has a slightly different preference in this regard. General recommendations include using a firm mattress and only one pillow. You don't want your head too flexed forward or extended while sleeping on your back. Ideally, your neck should be in the anatomic neutral position in order to wake up feeling rested and refreshed. We tend to prefer a high-quality memory foam mattress and pillow, such as those from Tempur-Pedic™. However, you might prefer another kind of mattress and pillow. If you select a spring mattress, look for one with a high coil count. The more coils in the spring, the firmer the mattress. As a general rule, if you purchase a full mattress, look for a coil count of 330 or greater. For a queen-sized bed, look for a coil count of 375 or greater. You don't want your mattress to be *too* firm. It should have a little give.

The best way to see if a mattress is right for you is to try it out in the store. Mattresses and pillows are not meant to last forever. If you haven't changed mattresses in more than 10 years, it's time to start looking for a new one.

The best position for your neck while sleeping is face-up on your back. If you like to sleep lying on your side, place a pillow between your knees. This will keep your spine in proper alignment, and it's good for your lower back as well as your neck. Lying on your stomach puts the most stress on your spine, so try to avoid this position.

5

Do It Yourself: Simple and Effective Exercises for Your Neck

In addition to helping you achieve good posture, exercises that stretch and strengthen your neck and upper back muscles can help take away your pain and keep it from coming back. Exercise is one of the most important investments you can make for the health of your neck. It's also one of the *easiest*. It doesn't require spending an hour at the gym. It doesn't even require expensive equipment—or much equipment at all! All you need is your upper back, neck, head, and arms, a Thera-Band®, and a long stick or ruler. Once your neck muscles are strong, relaxed, and well-balanced, good posture will be even easier to achieve and maintain.

> *Exercise is one of the most important investments you can make for the health of your neck.*

CHECK WITH YOUR DOCTOR FIRST

Before beginning any new exercise program, always check with your doctor about how much exercise you can safely perform. If at any time you develop chest pain, palpitations, headache, nausea, or vomiting while exercising, stop immediately and call your doctor.

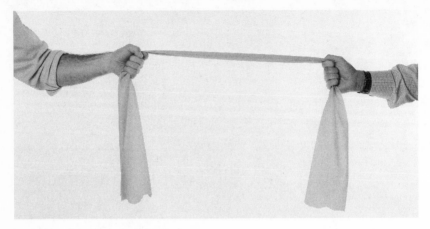

A Thera-Band® can be used for many exercises.

Thera-Bands® are available in any sporting goods store or on the Internet. If you don't have an elastic band, you can still do most of the exercises.

The last thing you will need is about 10 minutes of time to complete the workout.

Ready? Let's get started!

GENERAL EXERCISE PRINCIPLES

Let's review some general exercise principles:

1. Always make sure you continue to breathe throughout each exercise. One of the most common mistakes people make is to hold their breath while stretching and strengthening. It doesn't matter if you are an elite athlete, a weekend warrior, or a couch potato making a lifestyle change, holding your breath while exercising is counterproductive and dangerous. It can cause significantly elevated blood pressure, which, in turn, can lead to heart problems and a lack of oxygen flowing to your brain. Don't stress out about

your breathing—just remember to breathe slowly, calmly, and deeply throughout each exercise.

2. As a general rule, don't exercise through pain. Performing new exercises might be a bit uncomfortable at first, but they should *not* be painful. If you experience increased pain while performing any of the exercises in this book, stop and call your doctor.

3. An exercise program should have three components: aerobic, stretching, and strengthening. Because the exercise program in this chapter deals specifically with neck pain, we cover stretching and strengthening. Ideally, these exercises will not be the *only* ones you do during the day—you will also do a structured comprehensive program that includes stretching, strengthening, and aerobics.

> *An exercise program should have three components: aerobic, stretching, and strengthening.*

THE 10-MINUTE NECK EXERCISE PROGRAM: STRETCHING AND STRENGTHENING

This Neck Exercise Program can be done in about 10 minutes. You can do it in the morning before work, at your desk or during an office break, and/or before going to bed. Let's get started.

Exercise 1

This exercise has three parts:

A. Lie on your back, bend your knees so that your feet are flat on the ground, and extend your arms out to the side, as shown. Let the backs of your arms and hands fall to the ground in this position. Do not arch your back. Gently push the small of your back into the floor by tightening your abs at the same time as you relax your neck, chest, and upper back. Hold for 40 seconds.

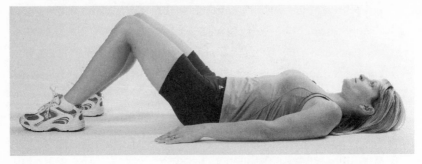

EXERCISE 1. A. Lie on your back, bend your knees until your feet are flat on the ground, then extend your arms to the side. Press the small of your back into the floor.

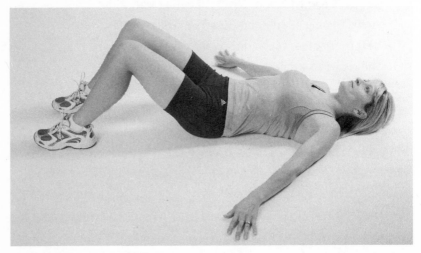

EXERCISE 1. B. Move your arms up 45 degrees and press the small of your back into the floor.

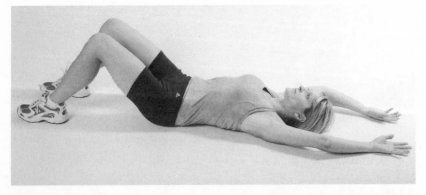

EXERCISE 1. C. Extend your arms above your head, press the small of your back into the floor and hold.

B. While still lying on your back, move your arms up 45 degrees and let them fall to the ground, as shown in the middle figure. Again, do not arch your back. Gently push your belly button into the floor as you relax your neck, chest, and upper back. Hold for 40 seconds. If you are able to do this comfortably, go to the next step. If it is difficult, take a 30-second break and then repeat this step. Do not go on until you can finish this step without difficulty.

C. While still lying on your back, extend your arms above your head and let them fall to the ground, as shown in the third part of the figure. Again, do not arch your back. Gently push your belly button into the floor at the same time that you relax your neck, chest, and upper back. Hold for 40 seconds.

Exercise 2

Sit in a chair, maintaining good posture. This includes sitting straight with your head above your neck (not flexed forward), abdominal muscles contracted, buttocks all the way back in the chair, and feet flat on the floor. Put your left hand, palm upwards, underneath your left buttock (so you are sitting on your hand). With your right hand, grab your left ear. Gently use your right hand to bring your head down toward your right ear. Hold this stretch for 30 seconds. Next, sit on your right hand (palm upwards), and with your left hand grab your right ear. Gently use your left hand to bring your head down toward your left ear. Hold this stretch for 30 seconds. Repeat this exercise two more times.

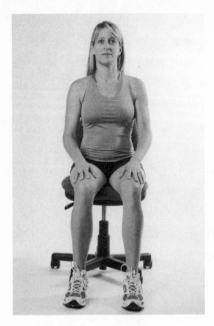

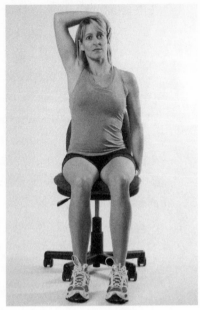

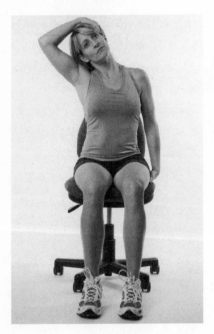

EXERCISE 2. Sit in a chair maintaining good posture. Next, place your left hand under your buttocks and grab your left ear with your right hand. Now, bring your head down toward your right ear; hold the stretch for 30 seconds. Repeat exercise 2 on the opposite side.

Exercise 3

Sit in a chair, maintaining good anatomic posture as in Exercise 2. Place your left hand, palm upwards, underneath your left buttock (so you are sitting on your hand). With your right hand, hold the back of the left side of your head, near your left ear. Gently use your right hand to bring your head down, so that you are looking toward your right hip. Hold this stretch for 30 seconds. Next, sit on your right hand (palm upwards), and with your left hand grab your right ear. Gently use your left hand to bring your head down, so that you are looking toward your left hip. Hold this stretch for 30 seconds. Repeat this exercise two more times.

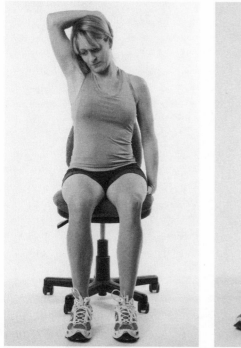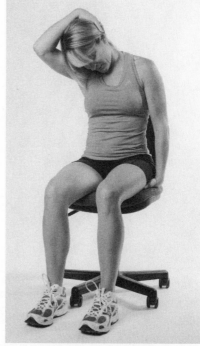

EXERCISE 3. Place your left hand underneath your left buttock and hold the back of the left side of your head with your right hand. Next, bring your head down to look toward your right hip; hold the stretch for 30 seconds. Repeat on the opposite side.

Exercise 4

Stand in good anatomic position, with your feet flat on the floor, weight on the balls of your feet, pelvis tucked under your spine (do this by squeezing your abdominal and gluteal muscles together), shoulders back and down, chest out, and with your head straight rather than flexed forward. With your hands behind your head and your fingers interlocked, gently bring your head downward, so that you are looking at your feet. Hold this stretch for 30 seconds. Repeat this exercise twice.

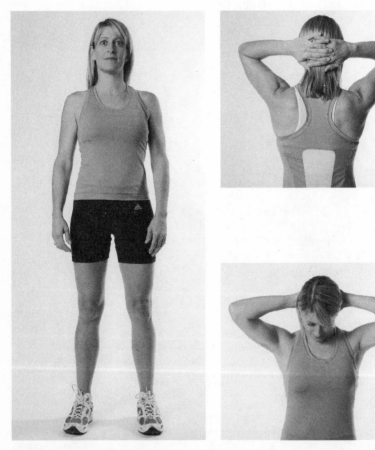

EXERCISE 4. Begin by standing in good anatomic position. Interlock your fingers behind your head. Then, bring your head downward; hold the stretch for 30 seconds.

Exercise 5

Still standing, place your right elbow and arm against a wall. Gently lean into your right arm in order to stretch your right chest muscles. Hold this stretch for 30 seconds. Next, repeat the exercise with your left elbow and arm against the wall, stretching your left chest muscles. Hold this stretch for 30 seconds. Repeat this exercise two more times.

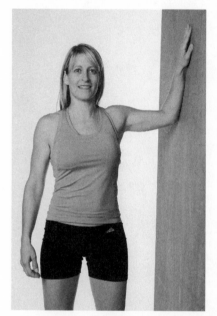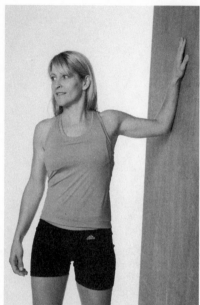

EXERCISE 5. Begin by placing your right elbow and arm against a wall. Then, lean into your arm to stretch the chest muscles; hold for 30 seconds.

Exercise 6

While still standing with your head perfectly straight above your spine, use your neck muscles to push your chin into your neck. Hold this position for 20 seconds. Rest for 30 seconds. Repeat two more times.

Exercise 7

Place the middle of a Thera-Band® in a closed door or wrap it around a door handle. With your arms extended (elbows flexed to about 10 degrees), hold onto the band. Without bending your arms, squeeze your shoulder blades together. Hold this position for 3 seconds. Slowly extend (relax) your shoulder blades. Without taking a break, repeat this contraction ten times. Take a 30-second break. Repeat two more times.

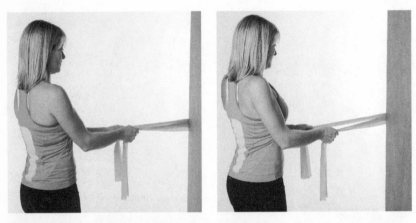

EXERCISE 7. Secure a Thera-Band® to a door. You can easily do this by tying a knot in the middle of the band and securely closing the door on the knot. Now, extend your arms and squeeze your shoulder blades together.

Exercise 8

Stand in front of the wall. Extend your arms (leaving only 2 or 3 degrees of flexion in your elbows) and place your palms on the wall so that you are leaning a bit on your arms. Push out against the wall, pushing through your palms so that your shoulder blades extend forward, as shown in the right part of the figure. Hold this position for 3 seconds. Slowly let your shoulder blades come back. Without taking a break, repeat this contraction ten times. *Don't push with your arms*—the force for this exercise should come from your ribs and under your scapula. Take a 30-second break. Repeat this twice more.

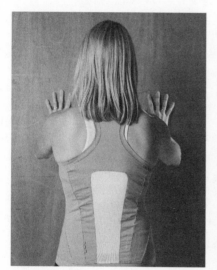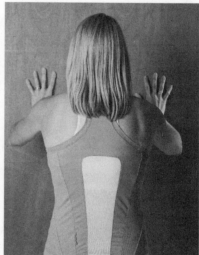

EXERCISE 8. Begin by placing your palms on the wall and leaning onto your arms. Then, push out against the wall so that your shoulder blades extend forward. Hold for 3 seconds, then slowly release.

If you do these exercises once or twice each day, your body and neck will thank you for it. These are the highest-yield exercises that you can do for your neck. They do not, of course, replace a complete, structured exercise program under the supervision of a physical therapist. The bottom line is that the healthier you stay overall, the healthier you'll feel and the less pain you'll have.

Aerobic exercise is also tremendously helpful for your overall health. Thirty to forty minutes of aerobic exercises four to seven times each week will benefit your entire body—especially your cardiovascular system—and help relax your muscles and improve the blood supply to the tissues of your neck.

Thirty to forty minutes of aerobic exercises four to seven times each week will benefit your entire body—especially your cardiovascular system—and help relax your muscles and improve the blood supply to the tissues of your neck.

One cautionary note about exercising applies to bicycling. Be careful not to hyperextend your neck while biking. Instead, ride your bike sitting up straight. A recumbent bike is also a good option. Swimming is an excellent exercise. However, if you're experiencing an acute episode of neck pain, don't use the crawl stroke that requires you to turn your head to the side to breathe. If you are a swimmer, and you can't wait to get back into the pool, do the crawl stroke while using a snorkel, so that you won't have to laterally rotate your neck in order to breathe.

Improving your posture and workstation, and doing these exercises will not return your neck to the way it felt when you were 15 years old, but it *will* help most people. If you implement these strategies and stick to your exercises, you have a good chance of staying pain-free. If these strategies aren't enough, others are available. We will explore them in the next two chapters.

TED AFTER EXERCISE AND POSTURE INTERVENTIONS

As we mentioned earlier, Ted was initially reluctant when we told him he needed to exercise. This wasn't because he didn't *want* to exercise—he just wasn't sure when he could find the time. Ted was naturally relieved when he saw how easy our exercise program was, and he committed to doing it twice a day—once in the late morning and again a few hours before the end of the work day. After one week of doing the exercises, he reported significant improvement in his pain.

Two weeks after starting the exercises, for the first time in months, Ted didn't notice his pain for *most* of the day. Inspired by the way he was feeling, he decided to dust off the treadmill in his basement. After putting his daughter to bed, he began going directly to the treadmill four times a week. He said it was a great way to meditate, work off some of the day's frustrations, and loosen up his muscles. Four weeks after improving his posture and workstation—and after implementing his new workout program—Ted happily and proudly reported a 98 percent improvement in his pain.

We couldn't have been happier for him. Ted will always need to be somewhat aware of his neck, but hopefully he won't have to experience the same level of pain again.

6

When Home Exercise Isn't Enough: It's Time to See the Doctor!

Most cases of neck pain are "benign," meaning that the source of the pain is a nonprogressive musculoskeletal problem. Put another way, the problem is an irritated muscle, ligament, tendon, or joint that does not require surgery and is *not* an infection or cancer. With this type of neck pain, it is reasonable to try some simple treatments that include improving posture and performing the simple exercises discussed in the last chapter.

It's time to see your doctor if neck pain significantly interferes with your life.

It's time to see your doctor if neck pain significantly interferes with your life, or if it doesn't improve after a week or two. You also need to see your doctor if you suspect a more serious problem, which might include an irritated nerve root in your neck that requires more urgent medical attention. Rarely, neck pain can be a sign of cancer, infection, or a spinal cord problem.

It is time to be concerned and seek medical attention if you experience any of the following symptoms:

▶ Your neck pain radiates down your arm.
▶ You experience numbness and/or tingling in your neck or arm(s).
▶ You experience weakness in your neck and/or arm(s).

▶ You have fevers and/or chills.

▶ The pain wakes you from sleep.

▶ You have night sweats.

▶ You experience unexplained weight loss or weight gain.

▶ You have an unexplained rash.

▶ You have been diagnosed as having rheumatoid arthritis.

▶ The pain does not improve after trying the postural interventions and exercises in the preceding chapters.

▶ The pain appears to have gotten worse over the past days or weeks.

It is important to emphasize that only a physician can offer you a diagnosis for *your* pain. You should speak with your doctor if you have any questions about pain, even if you don't have one of the above symptoms.

"Red Flag" Signs and Symptoms

Symptoms such as pain, numbness, tingling, or burning that radiates into your arm(s) might indicate that a nerve in your spine is being pinched or irritated. Weakness in your arm(s) might also indicate a pinched nerve. Fever and/or chills raise the red flag that an infection might be contributing to your pain. Unexplained weight loss, combined with neck pain, although rare, might indicate the presence of cancer. Likewise, pain that wakes you from sleep might indicate cancer. Rheumatoid arthritis can contribute to an unstable neck, because one of the ligaments (the *transverse ligament* at the *atlantoaxial joint* in the top of the cervical spine) tends to become loose. If you have rheumatoid arthritis and develop neck pain or other symptoms, always have it checked by your doctor. There are other explanations for these symptoms, but their presence makes it necessary to rule out the serious possibilities before we can be confident that the cause is benign.

What should you expect when you go to the doctor? First, as with Ted, she will probably begin with several questions about your pain, such as those listed below. If you plan to see your doctor, review these questions and consider what your answers might be. Make written notes to take with you to your appointment.

QUESTIONS THE DOCTOR MIGHT ASK ABOUT YOUR PAIN

▶ Where, exactly, are you experiencing pain?
▶ When did it start?
▶ Does it radiate down your arm?
▶ Do you have any numbness, tingling, burning, or weakness in your arm(s)?
▶ What makes the pain worse?
▶ What makes the pain better?
▶ What positions make the pain better or worse?
▶ What is your typical day like?
▶ Have you ever had a pain like this before?
▶ Did you ever experience a trauma to your neck?

Your doctor will also take a complete medical history, which might include asking such questions as:

▶ Do you have any medical problems, or have you had previous surgeries?
▶ Are you taking any medications?
▶ Do you have allergies?
▶ What are your social habits?
▶ Have you experiencing any recent new symptoms such as weight loss, fevers, or chills?

Next, the doctor will do a physical examination. When we initially examined Ted, we first evaluated the range of motion in his neck and arms. Then we tested his strength, sensation, and the reflexes in his arms. We *palpated* his neck (used our hands in a systematic way to feel), looking for, among other things, tightness, muscle spasms, and *trigger points*—muscle spasms that are painful and tender, and that also refer pain to areas that might not be directly over the spasm. Trigger points are essentially spasms of muscle that have referral pain patterns. We checked for other clinical signs in order to rule out other pathologies.

Unless there is a clinical suspicion of something unusual, such as an infection, blood tests are not generally necessary. Imaging studies, including an X-ray and possibly a magnetic resonance imaging study (an MRI), are more common.

X-rays are used primarily to evaluate bones. They are excellent for demonstrating certain problems, including fractures and bony mis-alignment. The major downside of an X-ray is that it involves radiation.

MRIs are excellent for evaluating soft tissues, such as interverte-bral discs and spinal nerves in the neck. They do not require radiation, but are much more expensive and take more time to perform. Open MRIs are available in most areas. The picture produced is usually ade-quate for most patients, and the open MRI is more easily tolerated by people who experience claustrophobia because there is more space inside the testing equipment.

After a comprehensive history and physical examination, and after any radiologic tests are done, you and your doctor should have a detailed discussion about your diagnosis and the treatment options.

TED'S CASE IN MORE DETAIL

Here is Ted's patient history from his first visit with us:

Chief Complaint:

Neck pain

History of Present Illness:

This is a 35-year-old man with an approximately 2-year history of chronic neck pain. He states that his pain is worse with range of motion, including rotation of his head from side-to-side. He does not recall exactly when the neck pain started, although it has been present for about 2 years, and he does not recall how it started. He denies any trauma to his neck or history of neck injury. He says that his neck is made worse by a long day at work or after sitting for a long period of time. He states that rest relieves his neck pain. He has taken over-the-counter pain relievers such as ibuprofen and Tylenol®, which help somewhat. At its worst, his neck pain can be as high as a 7/10 on the pain scale (where 0 is no pain, and 10 is worst pain imaginable). He has not seen a physician since his pain started.

Ted says that massage gives him some relief. Prior to the onset of his neck pain, he states that he was very active and pain-free. He even once completed a marathon. He is unable to participate in these activities now because of his pain, and he no longer goes to the gym or exercises at home. He says that his neck pain is making him "miserable" and even "a little depressed."

Past Medical and Surgical History

Ted has a history of seasonal allergies, and he had an appendectomy as a teenager. There is no history of significant trauma or prior neck injury.

Medications:

He takes ibuprofen and acetaminophen for pain, as needed. Claritin® as needed.

Allergies:

He has no known drug allergies.

Social History:

Ted is employed full-time at a financial firm. He works long hours and commutes up to 3 hours per day. During his work day, he might be sitting at his desk for extended periods of time, often up to several hours at a time. He does not leave the office during the day. He often works weekends. He does not smoke, and he drinks socially, up to several drinks per week. He is married and has two children, a 3-year-old daughter and a 7-year-old son.

Family History:

Ted's father is 70 years old and has been diagnosed with coronary artery disease. His mother is 65 years old and has been diagnosed with osteoarthritis of the knee. He has two siblings, a brother, 28 years old and healthy, and a sister, 31 years old and healthy, to the best of his knowledge.

Ted's maternal grandfather is elderly and has prostate cancer; his remaining grandparents are deceased; he does not know their cause of death.

Review of Symptoms:

- ▶ No radiating pain down one or both arms
- ▶ No numbness or tingling in the arms or hands
- ▶ No bowel or bladder dysfunction
- ▶ No difficulty with balance or walking
- ▶ No weakness in the arms or legs
- ▶ No fevers, chills, or night sweats
- ▶ No pain at night
- ▶ No progressive, worsening pain; Ted's pain is consistent and predictable

▶ There is no unintentional weight loss or gain. Ted notes a 10-pound weight gain over the last year. He attributes this to worsening eating habits and the fact that he no longer exercises regularly.

▶ No history of pain in the joints

▶ No skin rash or other skin problems

▶ No chest pain, shortness of breath, or abdominal pain

▶ No nausea, vomiting, or diarrhea

Physical Examination:

After gathering this valuable information, we examined Ted and found the following:

▶ His general appearance was good, and he did not appear to be experiencing great distress. We noted that he rubbed the back of his neck from time to time.

▶ His "vital signs" were: pulse: 70; blood pressure: 128/72; and respiratory rate: 12. These are all normal.

▶ Ted was able to flex and extend his neck, but had pain with both movements when he reached movement endpoints. He also had some discomfort when rotating his neck, but there was no significant loss of range of motion. The muscles of the back of the neck and over the upper trapezius muscles on both sides were tender to the touch. We also found several trigger points with referred pain patterns (pain that extends beyond the site at which you are pressing) in the trapezius muscles. There was no tenderness over the bones in the back of the neck, and no obvious abnormal positioning of the bones of the neck. There were no breaks in the skin.

▶ He had full strength in his arms and legs.

▶ He responded normally to both sharp and light touch in the upper and lower extremities.

▶ Reflexes in the upper and lower extremities were normal and symmetric—meaning they were the same on both sides.

▶ Ted walked with a normal gait pattern.

▶ We also did several tests to find out whether he might have nerve root compression in the neck and where the nerves exit the neck, none of which indicated any problem.

▶ Because his symptoms had been present for so long, we took X-rays to make sure that the bones looked good, and there were no surprises. The X-rays, as shown below, revealed a normal cervical spine, which is what we expected.

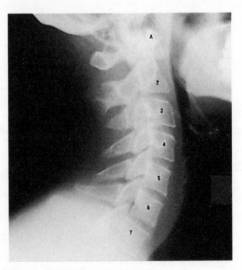

Ted's X-ray shows a normal cervical spine.

Our examination and tests confirmed the diagnosis we had suspected from his history and physical examination: chronic mechanical neck pain syndrome.

Before we proceed to a discussion of risk–benefit analysis in determining our treatment strategy for Ted, let's sum up the results of our history and physical examinations, and how they helped us to arrive at our diagnosis.

As we discussed earlier, we believed that Ted's chronic neck pain was most likely related to his poor habits. We explained earlier how his routine at work and home had contributed to his pain. Immobility, poor posture, and lack of sufficient movement and exercise had taken their toll on the supporting muscles, tendons, and ligaments of his cervical spine. Ted's history and physical examination supported our initial hypothesis and helped us rule out other possible causes for his pain. It also served to eliminate more ominous underlying disorders that can cause neck pain, such as rheumatoid arthritis and cancer.

How did we know these things? Each bit of information serves as a clue to solving the mystery of Ted's neck pain. First, the pain was localized to the back of his neck, and he did not have any pain, numbness, or tingling down his arms, which could be signs of nerve compression in the cervical spine. He also denied any weakness in the extremities, and he did not have any bowel, bladder, or balance problems, which would be symptoms of neurologic deficit. Since these were not present, we can be fairly certain that Ted has no "pinched nerves" or a spinal cord problem. The physical examination supported this conclusion, because Ted has full strength and sensation as well as normal reflexes in his arms and legs. He also had no difficulty with his balance when he walked. If Ted had a neurologic problem, at least one of these findings probably would have been abnormal.

The bones in the back of his neck were not tender on physical examination and his range of motion—while somewhat painful—was within normal limits. Based on these findings, we were able to conclude that there was no significant problem with the bones of Ted's neck, such as a fracture. Also, Ted denied having any "constitutional" symptoms— generalized abnormalities such as unintentional weight loss or weight gain, fever, chills, or night sweats that might lead us to suspect that a tumor or a systemic disease such as rheumatoid arthritis was causing his neck pain. With rheumatoid arthritis or other connective tissue diseases, Ted might have reported pain in other joints, or even skin problems such as a rash. However, he replied in the negative when asked about any history of such problems.

Finally, we ordered X-rays just to make sure the bones of Ted's neck were aligned and intact. X-rays helped confirm there was no fracture, misalignment, or significant arthritis to explain the symptoms. Typically, we order X-rays to *confirm* the tentative diagnosis we have already arrived at based on a person's medical history and physical examinations.

RISKS AND BENEFITS

Now, we are finally able to get to the essence of risk–benefit analysis, the key to choosing the right treatment. In Ted's case, this analysis was fairly straightforward. Given an initial diagnosis of previously untreated chronic neck pain, we prefer to start with a program of physical therapy. We also prescribe a home exercise program and educate the patient about how to change bad habits and practice good "neck hygiene." No medication was prescribed at the first visit, although we told Ted that he could take over-the-counter anti-inflammatory medication as needed. We preferred to first see how the therapy program would work. Although we suggested structured physical therapy with a therapist, Ted preferred to try the exercises on his own at first, because it was easier for him, given his busy schedule. Ted's symptoms were stable, and this was a reasonable compromise, so we agreed.

We already know the potential benefits of physical therapy, home exercises, and patient education, but we need to know the risks in order to complete the equation. Fortunately, there are relatively few risks to a properly prescribed physical therapy program. When we prescribe physical therapy, we include a diagnosis, directions about the therapy program, and any precautions that the therapist should keep in mind. Precautions are particularly important when there might be instability in the cervical spine—in patients with rheumatoid arthritis, for example. In people with heart or lung disease, the therapist needs to avoid over-working the patient, and should perhaps monitor blood pressure and oxygen levels in the blood. Ted is otherwise healthy and has a relatively uncomplicated neck problem, so there isn't too much to worry about in his case. As long as he is treated by an experienced and licensed physical therapist, the risk of side effects is very low. Given Ted's diagnosis, the potential benefits of physical therapy with patient education are high, and the potential for unwanted side effects is very low. Thus, we have an acceptable risk-to-benefit ratio, and can confidently and comfortably move forward with our prescription.

Because Ted wanted to do the exercises on his own at first, his increased risk factor is that he might not do the exercises in the proper way. We educated Ted extensively about the proper way to do the exercises, but it is still best to do them with a physical therapist on a regular basis. This way, if the exercise form starts to falter, the therapist is there to make the proper correction. We explained to Ted that if his symptoms did not get better, or if he experienced *any* increased pain while doing the exercises, he should stop and return for a follow-up visit. By ensuring that he would not exercise through pain, and that he would return if the exercises were not helping, we minimized any potential risks associated with his doing the exercises on his own.

Why didn't we prescribe any medication for Ted? A number of medications can be helpful for neck pain. However, all medications (including over-the-counter products) are associated with potentially significant side effects. We prefer to avoid medication, if possible. If we had prescribed a non-steroidal anti-inflammatory agent (NSAID), even one available over-the-counter, we would have put Ted at risk for stomach upset, possible ulceration or bleeding, or even kidney problems.

The risk for side effects increases significantly the longer any medication is taken.

The risk for side effects increases significantly the longer any medication is taken. This would certainly have negatively altered our risk-to-benefit ratio. Furthermore, we would have been unable to determine if physical therapy and patient education alone would alleviate Ted's neck pain. We can always add medication later, but the more conservative we can be in the beginning, the better. In Ted's case, this decision was the right one, and we were able to minimize his risk exposure.

People with neck pain who see their doctors need to remember that it is the physician's job to minimize the risk to them when recommending treatment. Usually, a physician will prescribe the most conservative treatment possible to achieve this goal. Keeping this in mind, if you see a physician for the first time because you have neck pain with no significant *neurologic deficits*—meaning numbness, tingling, weakness, progressive pain, change in bowel or bladder habits, or radiating pain—and she recommends that you undergo an epidural steroid injection or a surgical procedure, you should probably consider getting a second opinion.

What If Therapy Doesn't Work?

Everything seemed to work out for Ted. He did his home exercise program, improved his posture, and improved his ergonomics.

Ted got better—without medication and without injections or surgery.

We see this all the time, and we know that most patients improve with conservative treatment alone. But what if Ted hadn't made any progress? What if his neck continued to cause him pain and affect his life, despite our prescribed treatment? The next chapter offers further solutions.

7

Prescriptions for Conservative Care

For most people with "garden-variety" mechanical neck pain, like Ted, the interventions described in Chapters 4 and 5 are sufficient to take the pain away—and keep it away. However, they are not enough for 10–20 percent of the people with simple mechanical neck pain, and some people will require further medical evaluation and treatment. The good news for these people is that neck pain is one of the best-studied musculoskeletal problems, and effective treatments are *Neck pain is one of the best-studied musculoskeletal problems, and effective treatments are readily available.* readily available. In this chapter, and the two that follow, we'll describe all the tools your doctor has at his disposal to help you. We'll start with the most conservative ones. We'll also meet Sonia.

SONIA

Sonia's story was similar to Ted's. She is a 44-year-old corporate attorney, and she is married with two children. She works long hours, and when she came to see us she had been dealing with neck pain for almost a year. At first, she tried to simply ignore it. However, the pain had gotten worse over the last several months, and it was now interfering with her entire day. Her examination was also similar to Ted's. Like him, she opted to try exercising and improving her posture and ergonomics before starting a formal physical therapy program. We thought these interventions would help her, but we explained that if they didn't, the next step would be a structured course of physical therapy.

She returned after 4 weeks and said she felt about "20 percent better." Twenty-percent did not meet our expectations or—more importantly—Sonia's, so we started her on a structured course of physical therapy.

PHYSICAL THERAPY

Not all exercises are created equal. The exercises in this book are an excellent starting point, but nothing replaces a full physical therapy regimen supervised by a qualified therapist. Physical therapy is one of the most conservative and effective ways to treat many neck problems. In fact, most treatment approaches—even if they include medications, injections, or surgery—will *also* include physical therapy as the basis of the treatment.

Physical therapy has two primary components. The first is referred to as *passive,* because it emphasizes soft tissue massage, passive stretching, myofascial (muscle and fascial tissue) release, and modalities such as ultrasound, electrical stimulation, and ice and hot packs. This type of physical therapy is an excellent way to help calm down an acute flare or spasm of neck pain. It helps release the inflammation and break the cycle of pain. The second part of the therapy, which is often done in conjunction with the first, is the *active* part. This is when you can make lasting gains that will take your pain away and *keep it away.*

During the active part of therapy, you will work on strengthening your upper back and neck muscles, stretching your upper chest and neck, and on postural exercises. Many of these exercises are the same ones described in Chapter 5. However, the added benefit is that the therapist will give you hands-on active feedback about what you are doing right, and how you can improve your form. Your therapist will identify specific weaknesses and target them. Also, a typical therapy session lasts 40–60 minutes, so you will have more structured time to devote to your exercise program.

Your doctor and therapist will likely focus on other parts of your body that could be contributing to your pain. For example, because posture was particularly difficult for Sonia, we incorporated core strengthening into her exercise prescription. If a problem with the shoulder is contributing to the pain, exercises to stretch and strengthen the rotator cuff might be added.

Most of your time should be focused on the active part of your therapy. You will learn the exercises with your physical therapist, and then continue to do them on your own at home. This home exercise program begins while you are doing therapy, and continues once your formal therapy has ended. You might have only two to three physical therapy sessions each week, but you should do your exercises five times per week. A home exercise program is not much more intense than the exercises described in this book—and, in fact, ought to be very similar. The home exercise program should not take you more than 20–30 minutes. Once the exercises become easy for you, they can be done while you are at work or at home. We like to remind people that they can do their exercises in front of the television, and that they can be finished before the end of their favorite show!

SHOULD I WEAR A CERVICAL COLLAR?

Sonia asked us if she should wear a neck (cervical) collar, because her pain was significant. This is a good question, and we hear it a lot. There are many different types of cervical collars. The most common are the basic foam collars that you can purchase in a drugstore or medical supply store. But should you wear one?

The use of cervical collars by people with neck pain is controversial. Research suggests that the sooner the neck is *mobilized* (allowed to return to normal movement), the sooner the pain will be relieved; for example, such as after a whiplash injury resulting from a motor vehicle accident.

Even if there has been no specific injury to the neck, the sooner normal mobility is restored, the sooner the pain will get better. The problem with using a cervical collar is that you stop moving your neck, which might feel good temporarily, but it can lead to a tighter, stiffer neck in the long run. In essence, you can become dependent on a cervical collar—and ultimately have more pain even when using it.

The flip side to the argument against using a collar is that tight neck muscles that are in spasm need to rest and relax. A cervical collar can help provide this. Furthermore, when you are sleeping, the brain cannot tell the neck muscles to contract in ways that will keep your neck out of potentially painful positions the way it can during the daytime. This is why sometimes you wake up with a sore, aching neck. Wearing a cervical collar at night can help keep your neck from sliding into painful, awkward positions that would otherwise prolong your pain and inflammation. In addition, sleep is very important for healing, and it will be harder for your neck to heal if pain keeps you awake. If a cervical collar enables you to sleep, that's certainly a positive effect.

A Caveat to Cervical Collar Use

A cervical collar is *definitely indicated* if a person's neck is unstable—which might occur if there is a fracture, for example—or if there has been a significant trauma, and it is unclear whether or not the neck is stable. (Note that the words *stable* and *unstable* are used to indicate whether a spinal cord injury might result from the neck being unstable.) Over-the-counter foam collars are not sufficient to stabilize an unstable neck. A variety of collars are available that restrict neck movement to varying degrees, depending on the degree of instability and other factors.

With all this having been said, what should a person with neck pain do? Consider the following:

- ▶ Don't use a collar for more than 2 days without first checking with your doctor.
- ▶ Try to not use it for the entire day. Your neck needs movement. Make sure to move your neck through a comfortable range of motion. Do this gently if it's uncomfortable.

We prefer not to use cervical collars. When a patient has an acute spasm in the neck that is keeping her from sleeping, we *sometimes* suggest using a neck collar at *night only*—typically combined with a muscle relaxant. Movement is the key to restoring the neck to optimal health. Use a cervical collar with caution, and only when recommended by your physician.

Use a cervical collar with caution, and only when recommended by your physician.

Sonia was having trouble sleeping because pain occasionally woke her when she turned over. We told her to wear a soft cervical collar at *night only* for 1 week, while she started structured physical therapy. We also discussed different medications that might relieve her pain, but she did not want to take any medication.

Part III

Medical Solutions

8

Advanced Imaging Studies and Trigger Point Injections

SONIA'S FOLLOW-UP VISIT

Sonia returned 6 weeks after starting her formal physical therapy program. She had used the cervical collar for 1 week only while sleeping and then stopped, as we had previously agreed. She had gone to physical therapy and done her exercises consistently, but she reported only a 30 percent overall improvement.

"I did everything you said," she told us. "I went to all of my therapy sessions. I did everything the therapist wanted me to do. I did all of those silly exercises every day at home, and I totally changed the way I work—the way I sit at my desk, everything. And I only feel 30 percent better. Please don't make me do any more therapy!"

"Sonia," we said, "we're sorry to hear this. As you know, we were hopeful the therapy and exercises, and changing your habits would help. They usually do, but as we discussed, some people don't respond to these interventions. We might need to look at your neck in more detail with an MRI."

"What do you mean, doctor?" asked Sonia.

IMAGING STUDIES

Unfortunately, some people with neck pain do not respond to conservative treatment. In these cases, we usually want to look more closely at the anatomy of the person's neck. Typically, if someone still has significant

Some people with neck pain do not respond to conservative treatment.

pain after a course of conservative treatment, we consider ordering an MRI of the cervical spine. This allows us to look more closely at any anatomic abnormality that might be the person's "pain generator." As we discussed earlier, the intervertebral discs and facet joints within the cervical spine are among the usual "pain generating" suspects.

"Why didn't you just order the MRI when I was here the first time?" Sonia asked.

An MRI is a time-consuming and expensive test. It can also be uncomfortable for the patient to remain immobile in a confined space for up to an hour. Claustrophobia is a common complaint, and often people can't tolerate being inside the MRI machine for more than a few minutes. More importantly, most people with uncomplicated neck pain improve with conservative treatment and no imaging studies are needed—unless, of course, a "red flag" is found during the patient's history and physical examination.

We don't generally order these studies unless we want to rule out a more serious problem, or if we will change the treatment depending on the results. With Sonia, as with Ted, even if we saw arthritic facet joints or a bulging intervertebral disc, our initial treatment would have been the same—so there was no need for MRI at that time. Once someone like Sonia has not responded to physical therapy, however, we begin to consider possible injection procedures. Then it is reasonable and logical to obtain an MRI.

It is important to remember that findings on an MRI might or might not be correlated with symptoms; for example, many people with no pain have a herniated disc on MRI. Therefore, as we always tell our medical students and residents, you have to treat the patient, not the film.

WE TREAT PATIENTS, NOT MRIS

As doctors who treat pain, it is important to remember that the MRI is just one piece of the diagnostic puzzle. We must always bear in mind that the patient's history and physical examination are the real keys to making the correct diagnosis. Once we arrive at a diagnosis, we can apply our risk–benefit analysis and devise a treatment plan. In other words, we must never miss the "forest" for the "trees."

This orderly process is put at risk when a practitioner orders an MRI at the first hint of neck pain. The consequences can even be disastrous.

Here is an example of a patient whom we saw recently—the details and, of course, her name have been changed to protect patient confidentiality.

Sue came to our office with a 5-year history of neck pain. She did not have any history of radiating pain or weakness in her extremities. Nor did she report any "red flag" symptoms such as those we discussed earlier. Her neck pain was similar in many ways to Ted's and Sonia's. On her first visit to a "pain management" physician, she was prescribed an MRI of the cervical spine and given some pain medication. No physical therapy was prescribed, and there was no effort at patient education. During her follow-up visit a few weeks later, she was informed that she had a "herniated disc" in the cervical spine and that *cervical epidural steroid injections* would be helpful. A course of three consecutive injections was prescribed. After each of the injections, Sue had some relief of her pain, but it was short-lived.

Her physician then informed her that she was a "tough case," because her neck had failed to respond to conservative treatment. She was instructed to consult with a spine surgeon within the group. He told Sue told that surgery to the cervical spine would be her best chance of improving, although it could not be guaranteed.

Sue came to us for a second opinion prior to consenting to neck surgery. After evaluating her, we prescribed physical therapy, a home exercise program, and activity modification similar to Ted's. After about a month, she reported a 50 percent improvement in her pain. We then performed several trigger point injections. This resulted in further, lasting pain relief. At a follow-up appointment, she reported feeling about 80 percent better, and no further intervention was required. Although she was not pain-free, she was able to control her pain—the pain was *not* controlling her. Sue now understood the origin of her pain and had learned how to manage it. By being empowered in this way, she was able to return to activities that she had previously enjoyed, such as going to the gym and playing with her children.

What about that disc herniation? Was it contributing somehow to her pain? If so, to what degree? Or, was Sue's problem mostly due to soft tissue injury from poor mechanics and bad habits—what we call poor "neck hygiene?" Although the disc herniation might have played a role in her neck pain, a more conservative treatment approach was still indicated. If Sue's symptoms continued to bother her despite our best conservative efforts, and if her pain was disabling and significantly preventing her from doing the things she liked to do, we would have discussed surgical options.

An MRI can get you into tricky situations that you never anticipated. Therefore, we recommend the judicious and timely use of MRI. When the results are available, they should always be considered within the greater context of the patient's symptoms, signs, and findings on history and physical examination. In Sue's case, her disc herniation was obviously present on the MRI. However, it is up to the diagnostician to determine whether what is seen on MRI is the true cause of pain. Only when we treat the patient, and not the MRI, can we achieve this goal.

Of course, there *are* times when MRI is indicated sooner rather than later. Sometimes, an MRI is even indicated *immediately*. If a patient has any "red flag" symptom or sign, or has significant neurologic deficit—such as significant numbness or weakness—we will request an MRI immediately, because pathology might be present that requires immediate and aggressive attention. We also don't hesitate to refer our patients to surgical specialists in many of these cases.

We believe that injections within the cervical spine play an important role in pain control. They might be indicated when the patient is experiencing significant radiating pain, or when conservative care has truly failed.

Medial branch blocks are nerve block injections that are used to temporarily block pain signals coming from the facet joints in the neck. These blocks are used to evaluate whether the facets are causing the pain, and they are almost always indicated for chronic neck pain that does not respond to more conservative measures. We recommend surgical options for chronic neck only as a last resort because surgery involves the most risk. Typically, we advise a patient to consider surgery only after all other options have failed, including injections and medication.

> *An MRI can get you into tricky situations that you never anticipated. Therefore, we recommend the judicious and timely use of MRI.*

Sonia's Follow-Up Visit: Trigger Points

When we examined Sonia again, we again found several tender spots in the muscles of her lower neck and upper back. When we pressed on these points, Sonia experienced her typical neck pain. These are what we call *trigger points*.

Frequently, people with chronic neck pain have trigger points in the muscles of the upper back and neck. Trigger points often respond very well to physical therapy, exercise, postural improvements, and stretching. When this doesn't work, we recommend injecting the trigger points to "reset" the muscle and break the cycle of spasm and pain. Trigger point injections are made into the muscle only and involve significantly less risk than a spinal injection. However, any time you perform an injection of any type, there is always a risk of infection, bleeding, and/or damage to the structures through which the needle will pass. Although these risks are very low when the procedure is performed correctly, they still must be considered. Remember that risks are *always* associated with the potential benefits of any medical intervention.

Trigger point injections can be done with only a needle (no medication is injected), with lidocaine (an anesthetic like the one your dentist uses), or with lidocaine *and* steroid. Of course, the less medication injected, the less aggressive the procedure. If steroid is used, side effects from the steroid itself can occur, including temporary facial redness and flushing, prolonged bleeding during a women's period for one cycle, a temporary increase in blood sugar, irritability, and skin discoloration and atrophy. Multiple trigger point injections can be performed during the same office visit.

> *Risks are always associated with the potential benefits of any medical intervention.*

Research does not support one type of trigger point injection over another. In our opinion, it is much more important to get accurate *placement* of the injection, as opposed to *what* is injected. The most important point of a trigger point injection is to inject directly into the epicenter of the trigger, in order to break up the spasm. When this is done correctly, a classic "twitch" is produced in the muscle, followed by an immediate release of muscle tension. Pain relief is sometimes immediate, and it might range from 1 to 100 percent. In some cases, it takes a day or two for the pain to subside. Steroids can take 3–7 days to have an effect—and the pain might not completely subside until a week or two later. Placing a bag of ice (or frozen peas) for 15 minutes on the injection(s) site the night of the injection can help minimize any post-injection bruising.

BOTULINUM TOXIN (BOTOX®, MYOBLOC®) INJECTIONS

Another way to relieve trigger points and tight muscles is with *botulinum toxin*, most commonly referred to as Botox®, although there are multiple forms of botulinum toxin. Botox® is the brand-name drug; the generic medication is botulinum toxin type A. Botulinum toxin type B is prescribed under the trade name Myobloc®. There are subtle differences between Botox® and Myobloc®, and research is ongoing to determine which toxin might be the most appropriate for which indications. Botulinum toxins, as a group, have received increasing interest and have been applied to a wide variety of disorders.

Botulinum toxin is essentially a muscle relaxant. Its best known use is in a cosmetic procedure to remove wrinkles, which are the result of small contractions of the muscles in the skin. Injecting Botox® into the skin inhibits these contractions, causing the wrinkles to disappear. Similarly, when injected into trigger points in the neck, Botox® or Myobloc® can relieve muscle spasms.

Botulinum toxin for neck pain is an *off-label* use of the drug, meaning that the Federal Drug Administration (FDA) has not approved its use for neck pain. This does *not* mean that the FDA has said it *can't* be given for this purpose, but rather that not enough research has been done to allow the FDA to validate this specific usage. Research needs to be done to understand exactly which patients with chronic neck pain, if any, might benefit from botulinum toxin injections. At present, these injections should be reserved for patients with pain that is resistant to other more conventional therapies, and the patient should clearly understand that no research definitively supports its usage. The case can even be made that if *too much* botulinum toxin is injected, the protective features of the neck muscles might be compromised, and further damage might be done to the underlying structures. In the coming years, hopefully sufficient research will be reported, so that we can better advise whether this is a worthwhile treatment.

One final note on botulinum toxin treatment for neck pain: Some insurance companies cover it, but others do not. If it is not covered by your insurance, it's a costly proposition. One vial of Botox® is typically used, and it can cost close to $600. Myobloc® is not used as often, but it might be less expensive.

SONIA'S TRIGGER POINT INJECTIONS

We identified three trigger points in Sonia's neck that seemed to be causing most of her pain. After talking about the pros and cons of the injection, we obtained informed consent to perform the trigger point injections. We did them using 1-percent lidocaine. We prefer not to use steroid in our trigger point injections except in rare instances, and we are very careful to make sure our injections are placed in the correct anatomic location within the muscle.

Sonia responded very well to the injections. Immediately afterwards, she reported almost 95 percent pain relief. Because her pain was almost completely resolved, we did not order an MRI. If her pain had returned, we would have reviewed her situation again, and we might have ordered an MRI.

We advised Sonia that the pain relief obtained from the injections might not last. The best way to make sure the positive results would persist was for her to continue with her home exercise program and the improved posture she had learned. In essence, the injections offered a "window of opportunity" during which she could take advantage of the pain relief in order to alter her biomechanics and prevent her pain from returning.

9

Medications for Neck Pain

It is important to understand that no medication can *cure* your neck pain. Talk with your doctor before you take any medication for pain. Before we discuss the medications that you can take by mouth, we'll cover *topical medications*—those that are absorbed through the skin.

TOPICAL MEDICATIONS

In general, we advocate trying topical creams and sprays before using oral medications, because topical medications are applied locally and diffuse through the skin to the area of pain and inflammation. Therefore, the *systemic absorption*—the amount of medication that gets into the bloodstream and is distributed throughout the body—and thus the side effects, are generally much less. If you take a medication by mouth, it has to pass through your stomach, intestines, liver, kidneys, and bloodstream before reaching the painful region of your neck. In the process, the medication will reach every other part of your body as well.

Talk with your doctor before you take any medication for pain.

It is important to realize two things about topical medications. First, they *are* medications. As such, they must be used with appropriate caution and only as directed. Second, although topical medications are excellent for *superficial* joints—joints that are close to the skin, such as those of the hands and ankles—they might not diffuse into the deeper structures in the neck. Nevertheless, they are an appropriate first-line medication to try.

Common over-the-counter topical pain relievers include Capzasin-P® cream, Ben-Gay®, and Icy Hot®, to name just a few. Three that are available only by prescription include topical lidocaine 5-percent patches (Lidoderm®), topical diclofenac (Voltaren®), and topical diclofenac epolamine patches (Flector®).

The topical Lidoderm® patch contains a *topical anesthetic* that diffuses through the skin and numbs the underlying soft tissues. These patches are generally very well tolerated but do not address any underlying inflammation. The anti-inflammatory medication in the topical patches containing Voltaren® diffuses through the skin to reduce inflammation. The advantage of taking anti-inflammatory medication by patch or gel, instead of orally as a pill, is that much less of the medication actually reaches the bloodstream. As a result, the potential for side effects—although still present—is substantially reduced.

ORAL MEDICATIONS

Three broad classes of medications are available for neck pain: anti-inflammatories, pure analgesics ("painkillers"), and muscle relaxants.

The most common types of oral anti-inflammatory medication are nonsteroidal anti-inflammatory drugs (NSAIDs). You will recognize them by their names: ibuprofen (Advil® and Motrin®), naprosyn (Aleve®), acetylsalicylic acid (aspirin), diclofenac (Voltaren®), and indomethacin (Indocin®), to name a few. These medications all work in approximately the same way—by blocking enzymes (proteins in your body) that create inflammation. Their advantage is that they address the inflammatory as well as pain component of your neck symptoms. However, because they are taken orally, the medication spreads throughout your body, and only a small amount reaches the site of inflammation in your neck. Still, they can be very helpful for certain cases of neck pain.

Side effects are a major downside of NSAIDs. These are *not* benign medications. They are believed to be responsible for as many as 200,000 hospital admissions per year, and up to 20,000 deaths. Common side effects include stomach and kidney problems. NSAIDs raise your blood pressure and can result in heart attack or stroke. Although there is a role for NSAIDs in the treatment of some cases of neck pain, they should be taken with caution and only when necessary.

COX-2 inhibitors are a newer type of NSAID, available only by prescription. These medications specifically target an enzyme (cyclooxygenase; COX) that is involved in the development of inflammation. Initially, it was thought that by being more specific, they would have fewer side effects. The COX-2 inhibitors Vioxx® and Bextra® were withdrawn from the market because of cardiovascular side effects and a rare dermatologic side effect in Bextra®. Celebrex®, another COX-2 inhibitor, remains on the market, but it also has potential side effects similar to NSAIDs.

The steroid *prednisone* is the most potent oral anti-inflammatory agent currently available. However, oral prednisone is associated with side effects that can include mood changes, irritability, insomnia, facial flushing and sweating, increased blood pressure, weight gain, osteoporosis, increased susceptibility to infections, changes in menstruation, and adrenal shock—to name just a few. Long-term oral steroid use is not indicated for the treatment of isolated neck pain. However, a short (5-day) treatment with steroids is sometimes used. This is generally well-tolerated, although not always. Because the medication is taken orally and thus affects the entire body, using it—even for a short period of time—is reserved for severe cases when no better alternative is available.

PAIN MEDICATIONS

Analgesics ("painkillers") are another broad class of medication. The most common of these is acetaminophen (Tylenol®), which is primarily a pain reliever. It can be a very effective weapon against pain. Great care must be taken to not overdose on acetaminophen, which is also an active ingredient in other over-the-counter medications, such as drugs for headache, colds, and the flu. Never take more than four grams of acetaminophen in a day—and if you do take it, don't drink alcohol, because the combination can potentially result in liver failure and death.

Tramadol (Ultram®) is another pain medication that is available only by prescription. It acts in a different way than acetaminophen. Tramadol is similar to narcotic medications and has an effect on the same opiate receptors as narcotics, but it is not as addictive as narcotics—or as effective at relieving pain. If you are taking antidepressants or muscle relaxants, you should not take tramadol as this combination might result in a seizure. Its most common side effects include dizziness, drowsiness, gastrointestinal upset (nausea, constipation, and vomiting), and insomnia. Before taking any new medication, be sure discuss the pros and cons with your doctor, including potential interactions with any other medications you might be taking.

Never take more than 4 grams of acetaminophen in a day—and if you do take it, don't drink alcohol, because the combination can potentially result in liver failure and death.

The next step up the pain medication ladder is narcotic agents. Narcotics are excellent painkillers, and they can be either short- or long-acting, so one can be selected based on the type and extent of pain, but major issues are associated with them. Narcotic medications can be addicting, and they can cause constipation and sleepiness. Despite their potential side effects, narcotics are sometimes indicated for patients with acute episodes of particularly severe neck pain.

Muscle Relaxants

Often, muscle spasm is a contributing factor in neck pain, and sometimes it's the true underlying cause. For this reason, muscle relaxants are another class of oral medications used to treat neck pain. A muscle that is fatigued from constantly being strained all day in a suboptimal anatomic position often responds by going into spasm—whether this is caused by bad posture, a poorly set-up workstation, and/or tight or weak muscles. Also, if an underlying nerve, joint, or ligament is injured, the overlying muscle might go into spasm in a counterproductive measure to "protect" the underlying structures. Of course, this spasm just perpetuates the pain—plus the spasm itself is typically painful.

Muscle relaxants are prescription medications. Side effects are common and include drowsiness. During an acute episode of neck pain, it is sometimes reasonable to use a low-dose muscle relaxant at night to help your muscles relax and let you fall asleep.

An Important Note about Medications

As we discussed earlier, medications don't cure neck pain. They can help to manage pain and—to a certain degree—inflammation. When should drugs be taken for neck pain? Ideally, they should be reserved for times when the neck pain is significant. When medications *are* used, they should be considered a *bridge* that will allow you to do your exercises and recover from an acute flare-up of pain—so you can get back to your life and into doing your exercises. Medications present a *window of opportunity* that can help you get back to your exercise regimen. Your exercises and improved posture will keep you pain-free in the long run. If you find yourself taking medications for more than a month, even if it's an over-the-counter medication, such as acetaminophen or ibuprofen, stop and reassess your situation with your doctor—there is probably something more you can do.

X-Ray-Guided Injections and Surgery

Every patient is different, and a wide range of opinion exists among doctors when it comes to selecting the best treatment for any specific condition. The medications and other treatments we have discussed so far might be prescribed at any point during the course of treatment, depending on the physician's best judgment. As we discussed earlier, it is the physician's job to design a treatment plan that minimizes risk at the same time that it maximizes the potential for benefit. We prefer to climb the risk ladder incrementally and to keep our prescribed treatments as simple and as targeted as possible. To us, the key is always diagnosis, diagnosis, diagnosis. The rest flows from there.

SEAN'S NECK PROBLEMS

Sean's situation was very similar to that of Ted and Sonia. Sean is a 44-year-old investment banker who works long hours, is married, and has four children. He differed from Ted and Sonia in that he did not respond to exercise, postural adjustments, ergonomic interventions, or trigger point injections. We also prescribed a muscle relaxant medication to be taken at night, but his pain persisted.

When Sean came for his third follow-up appointment, it was clear that he was frustrated. He often told us, "I don't have time for this pain."

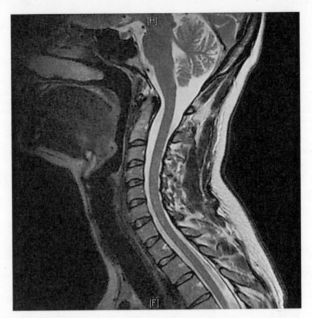

MRI of Sean's cervical spine. Courtesy of radswiki.net.

We ordered an MRI of his cervical spine, so that we could review the film during his next appointment. Sean's film can be seen above.

His MRI revealed good spinal alignment, no intervertebral disc bulges, and mild arthritis of the lower cervical facet joints. Given Sean's history of a motor vehicle accident when he was in his 20s, and the fact that there was some arthritis in his facet joints, we decided to focus on these joints as the potential cause of his pain.

Facet Joint Pain

As we noted earlier, facet joints are the small joints in the back of your spine. They permit flexion and extension of the neck, and they resist rotation. Facets joints are the most common cause of chronic neck pain. If you have a history (even remote) of a car crash or other trauma to your neck—but even if you haven't—your facet joints might be the cause of your neck pain. If your pain persists for longer than 3 months, despite aggressive conservative care, the facet joints might need to be considered as the potential culprit.

There are two ways to accurately diagnose facet joints as being the cause of neck pain. Both involve injecting in or around the joints using an X-ray to guide accurate needle placement. In one injection technique, the joints themselves are injected with anesthetic and steroid. This injection involves penetrating the joint capsule. The injection itself is diagnostic—if it takes away the pain, the pain generator might have been found. The advantage of this type of injection is that the steroid has the potential to have a therapeutic effect as well as a diagnostic effect. The disadvantage is that some of the medication might leak out (if there is a torn joint capsule) and spread. If this happens, the diagnostic aspect of the test can be compromised because the medication might, in fact, be treating an adjacent structure in the neck.

Facets joints are the most common cause of chronic neck pain.

The other injection procedure involves injecting anesthetic medication only. This is called a *medial branch block*. The medial branch of the *dorsal ramus* innervates the facet joint. By anesthetizing it, the facet joint can no longer communicate the sensation of "pain" to the brain. The advantage of this type of injection is that it is very precise. If it takes away your pain, we are much more confident that the facet joint is indeed the source of your pain. The disadvantage of this type of injection is that it is *only* diagnostic, and the anesthetic wears off after a few hours. However, arriving at a diagnosis is a major key—particularly if we find that the facet joints are the cause—because very good treatment is available.

To be sure that we don't receive false-positive results from the medial branch block injection, we need to perform two injections, with anesthetics of different durations or time of action. One uses lidocaine, a short-acting anesthetic. The other, which is done on a different day, uses bupivacaine, a longer-acting anesthetic. In some cases, neither the physician doing the injection nor the patient knows which anesthetic is used for each injection until both blocks are performed. For practical reasons, in many cases the physician does know which anesthetic is used in which block, but the patient does not.

In either case, a positive test result is confirmed when the patient reports having longer pain relief with the longer-acting anesthetic than with the shorter-acting one. Performing the injections in this way vastly reduces the number of false-positive blocks (the chance for the patient response be due to a placebo response), and it means that the physician and patient can be confident that the facet joint(s) in question is indeed the cause of pain.

SEAN'S FACET JOINTS

We discussed with Sean the pros and cons of medial branch block injections. We explained to him that if we were able to diagnose his facet joints as the source of his pain, the next step would be to "burn" or "sever" those nerves using radiofrequency energy. This procedure is called *radiofrequency neurotomy*. If the facet joints are the pain generator, this procedure will semi-permanently block the pain signals from these joints and thus alleviate the pain. It is only "semi-permanent" because the nerves slowly regenerate. Pain relief will typically last from 6 to 12 months. When/if the pain returns, the procedure can be repeated. In some patients, for whatever reason, the pain never returns.

Following our recommendation, Sean decided to proceed with the medial branch blocks. We did four injections (two medial branches supply each facet joints) on two different days with different duration-acting anesthetics. He had 100 percent pain relief following both sets of injections, and the relief lasted longer with bupivacaine than with lidocaine. Therefore, we were confident that Sean's lower cervical facet joints were the cause of his pain. We scheduled him for radiofrequency neurotomy of the medial branches that had been tested.

RADIOFREQUENCY NEUROTOMY

Radiofrequency neurotomy is a *percutaneous* procedure—meaning it is done with needles through the skin. The skin is not cut and sutures are not required.

The procedure has an excellent success rate when done on the right patients, which are those who have at least 80–90 percent pain relief from anesthetic injections, and who experience longer relief from the longer-acting anesthetic.

As with other injection procedures, radiofrequency neurotomy should be coupled with addressing the underlying biomechanical issues. Sean had an excellent response to the radiofrequency neurotomy. He reported 100 percent pain relief 4 weeks after the procedure—it takes about that long for complete healing from the procedure. We explained to Sean that although we were very happy for him, his pain might return in 6 months to a year, and that we could repeat the procedure if this happened. However, the best way to ensure that his pain did *not* return was to correct his posture and workstation, and continue his home exercise program.

EPIDURAL STEROID INJECTIONS

Epidural steroid injections are done with X-ray (fluoroscopic) guidance into the *epidural space* near the spinal cord. This term describes a space within the spinal canal that is *epi*, meaning *outside* of the dura, a tissue that surrounds the spinal cord and spinal nerves. When done by an experienced clinician, these injections are relatively safe. However, they have been known to cause spinal cord damage, paralysis, and even death. Cervical epidural steroid injection should only be done when absolutely necessary. This type of injection should *not* be done in cases of straightforward acute neck pain.

Conditions for which epidural injections are appropriate include a pinched nerve or nerves in the neck that do not respond to conservative care, an irritated cervical intervertebral disc that is not responding to more intensive conservative measures, and radiating symptoms of pain, numbness, and/or tingling down the arm that does not respond to conservative care.

Cervical epidural steroid injection should only be done when absolutely necessary.

As with the management strategies discussed earlier, any injection procedure or medication will work best when coupled with a proper exercise regimen, improved posture, and improvements in workstation set-up and ergonomics.

SURGERY

Surgery involving the neck is a very serious matter, to say the least. However, surgery is clearly indicated for some patients and conditions. For example, someone with new bowel and bladder incontinence and profound weakness—and who is found to have a herniated disc that is causing spinal cord compression—is a candidate for emergency surgery. Other people are clearly not surgical candidates, but they only *think* they are.

DON'S NECK PAIN

One patient who came to us for a surgical opinion was a 31-year-old man with a 6-year history of neck pain. Don had been to several doctors. He had received chiropractic manipulations, physical therapy, trigger point injections, epidural steroid injections, facet injections, and now he was considering surgery. He wanted an opinion about whether he should see a neurosurgeon. He didn't have any symptoms in his arms or neurologic findings. Don's MRI revealed some mild degenerative changes, but nothing that would explain his pain. We asked this otherwise healthy young man why he was considering asking a surgeon to cut his neck open and dig around in his spine.

"Maybe they'll see something—maybe they will see what is causing my pain," was his reply.

We understood Don's frustration. He had pain and had been looking ardently for a cure. We also appreciated the sentiment that if a surgeon can just "take a look inside," she will be able to "see" the problem. Trust us—*nothing* has a greater potential for disaster than a surgeon doing surgery for isolated neck pain when nothing on the imaging studies is shown to be causing the pain.

Surgery is definitely not the right option if there is no clear lesion on MRI, computed tomography (CT), X-ray, or other imaging modality, and if there are no neurologic signs or symptoms. Signs and symptoms that might indicate surgery *is* appropriate include progressive numbness, weakness, and/or bowel/bladder changes. However, even in the face of these symptoms, if no lesion was present on imaging studies that could be surgically addressed, it is unlikely that surgery would be appropriate.

Things get a bit more complicated when someone has a *high intensity zone* that indicates inflammation in a bulging cervical disc, and all signs point toward it as the cause of pain. In this case, *cervical discography* can be performed to confirm that the disc is the cause of pain. This is an invasive test that involves inserting a needle into the intervertebral disc in the neck, injecting a contrast dye, and seeing if it reproduces the patient's pain. If cervical discography confirms that the disc is the source of neck pain, cervical fusion might be an appropriate option. This remains a controversial topic that must be addressed on a case-by-case basis.

> Nothing *has a greater potential for disaster than a surgeon doing surgery for isolated neck pain when nothing on the imaging studies is shown to be causing the pain.*

WHAT HAPPENED TO DON?

After spending some time with Don, we learned two surprising things about his case. First, no one had ever evaluated his workplace or talked with him about biomechanics. Don is a corporate lawyer. He had been given a headset to use instead of a handheld phone, but his computer was badly positioned for his body. His hands had to reach too far forward for the computer and his head slumped forward. His positioning resembled Ted's as shown on page 39.

The second surprising thing about Don was that, although he had gone through 3 months of physical therapy, the therapy had been 4 years ago, and he had not been taught an exercise regimen. We sent him to a physical therapist to work on his posture and focus on strengthening his rhomboids and trapezius and stretching his pectoral muscles. We also did trigger point injections into his trapezius muscle.

After 3 weeks, he reported feeling 20 percent better than he had felt in years. We identified more trigger points in his rhomboid major and injected them. He continued with his therapy and also improved his workstation ergonomics and posture. Three weeks later he reported a 50 percent improvement. We didn't find any additional trigger points. We discussed the possibility of medial branch blocks to evaluate whether the facet joints were contributing to his pain. However, Don was happy with his progress and wanted to continue with what he was doing. This seemed reasonable to us.

He finished his therapy and continued with his home exercise program of stretching and strengthening exercises. At our suggestion, he also started going with his wife for a brisk 30-minute walk each evening. We didn't hear back from Don until about a year and a half later, when he injured his lower back playing football with his kids in the backyard. We asked him how his neck was doing.

"I meant to send you a card," Don said. "My neck is almost normal. It still acts up sometimes when I don't do my exercises, but then I start doing them again and the pain goes away. It's amazing how simple it was to fix my neck pain. Thank God I didn't get the surgery! I can't thank you enough."

Medications and injections are important in the treatment of some cases of neck pain, but they *never* take the place of the treatment basics. In our experience, when someone has had neck pain for awhile and has been bouncing from one doctor to another, often we find that the basics have been overlooked. As we tell our medical students and residents, always remember the basics and work up from there.

Medications and injections are important in the treatment of some cases of neck pain, but they never take the place of the treatment basics.

Part IV

Alternative and Complementary Solutions

11

Supplements

If you have an ache, ailment, cramp, worry, concentration problem, hair loss, or other trouble…and certainly if you are concerned about sexual performance—don't worry—someone wants to sell you a supplement! Do they work? More importantly for this book, do any of them work for neck pain?

Despite the prevalence of neck pain, supplement manufacturers have been relatively slow to target this potential market. However, numerous supplements are marketed for arthritis and general "pain conditions," and the argument can readily be made that neck pain often falls under both categories.

GLUCOSAMINE AND CHONDROITIN SULFATE

Two supplements that have received the most attention for treating arthritis are glucosamine and chondroitin sulfate. They can be purchased either separately or together in a combined supplement. The essential rationale for their use is that they are believed to help restore the natural cartilage in joints in a variety of ways. Cartilage is an essential substance in most joints, including your knees, hips, shoulders, ankles—and facet joints. They don't look the same, and they are a lot smaller, but the truth is that the small facet joints in your back are very similar to your knee joints. If a substance really could increase the amount of healthy cartilage in your facet joints without causing side effects, it would be worth taking. But, the important question is whether a substance has yet been found that can do this.

Many studies published in prestigious medical journals have strongly advocated the use of glucosamine and chondroitin sulfate in the treatment of arthritis of the knee. Recent studies have started to question whether the conclusions of the earlier studies were hastily drawn or misguided. Nevertheless, given the relative absence of side effects—except the impact on your wallet, which is not trivial and can be as much as $300–$400 per year—it is more than reasonable for people with arthritis of the knee to consider trying glucosamine and chondroitin sulfate to lessen their pain, and possibly even restore cartilage growth. What about other forms of arthritis? For a complete discussion of these supplements, see *The Arthritis Handbook: Improve Your Health and Manage the Pain of Osteoarthritis* by Grant Cooper, M.D.

The real question is, "Should you take glucosamine and chondroitin sulfate for neck pain?" If the pain in your neck is largely muscular, glucosamine/chondroitin sulfate supplements are unlikely to be helpful. If, however, poor biomechanics in your neck muscles has led to repetitive stress and strain on the facet joints in your back, causing arthritis in them, glucosamine/chondroitin might be worth trying in conjunction with postural re-education and exercise.

If you have experienced neck pain for more than 3 months and have not started treatment, it is reasonable to take supplements in conjunction with the recommendations in the first chapters of this book.

If you have experienced neck pain for more than 3 months *and* have not started treatment, it is reasonable to take supplements in conjunction with the recommendations in the first chapters of this book. After 3 months, if you are feeling better, stop taking the glucosamine/chondroitin. If the pain returns despite continuing your exercise regimen, start taking them again. If the pain does not return, don't take

> ### AN IMPORTANT POINT ABOUT GLUCOSAMINE AND CHONDROITIN SULFATE
>
> If you decide to take glucosamine and chondroitin sulfate, it is important to know that, as of the time of this writing, *there is no evidence in the medical literature to support its efficacy for treating neck pain*. This does not mean that you should not take it. There are many medical treatments that have not been fully studied, and which we do not completely understand. The bottom line is that a treatment might be worth trying if there is a good scientific rationale for why it might/should work, if the side effects are minimal, and if the potential gains are significant. The rationale for using glucosamine and chondroitin sulfate, as previously discussed, is that it has been shown to help restore joint health in knees. Therefore, it is not unreasonable to believe that it might help restore the health of the spinal facet joints.

them again. Just realize that we'll never know for sure whether the supplements were helpful in decreasing your pain or not. The bottom line is that your pain is better.

HOW TO TAKE GLUCOSAMINE AND CHONDROITIN SULFATE

Because supplements are not regulated by the Food and Drug Administration (FDA), and because of the difficulty in regulating the multi-billion dollar supplement industry, what a manufacturer claims is in the bottle might or might not really be in the bottle. Studies have shown that more than half of glucosamine supplements do not contain the amount of glucosamine claimed on the label. Be sure to buy from a reputable dealer who has been in business for awhile.

If you are pregnant, thinking of becoming pregnant, nursing, or under the age of 18, do not take glucosamine and/or chondroitin without first talking to your doctor.

The dosages that have been studied the most for osteoarthritis of the knee include 1,600 mg of chondroitin sulfate and 1,800 mg of glucosamine sulfate. These are reasonable dosages to try for chronic neck pain as well. If there is no improvement after 3 months, it is advisable to stop taking the product.

The most common side effect of these supplements is a mildly upset stomach. If this or any other adverse reaction occurs, stop taking the product and contact your doctor. If you are pregnant, thinking of becoming pregnant, nursing, or under the age of 18, do not take glucosamine and/or chondroitin without first talking to your doctor.

> ### BE CAUTIOUS IF YOU ARE ALLERGIC TO SHELLFISH
>
> Glucosamine is made from the protein in the shells of shellfish. If you have a shellfish allergy, talk to your doctor before taking the supplement. Although no shellfish should be in the supplement, theoretically contamination during the manufacturing process could cause problems. "Shellfish-free" glucosamine products are available. Talk to your doctor about the option that is right for you.

SAM-E

S-adenosylmethionine (SAM-e) has been available by prescription for some time in Europe for the treatment of depression and osteoarthritis. In the United States, it is considered a dietary supplement. The plus side of this designation is that it is available over-the-counter at your local drugstore in the United States. On the downside, the quality of the product will not be guaranteed by the FDA, and what is advertised might or might not be what you get. As with any supplement, make sure you buy from only the most reputable manufacturers.

SAM-e is a synthetic form of a naturally occurring substance in the body that is involved with more than 30 biochemical processes. It is believed to potentially improve cartilage (that crucial component of facet and other joints), as well as improve depression.

People with neck pain are not inherently depressed. However, neck pain—or chronic pain of any kind—*can* take its toll on the psyche. Additionally, the added stress of dealing with chronic pain is often carried—you guessed it—in those very same tight muscles and shoulders that caused the pain in the first place. Clearly, this sets up a potentially difficult cycle of pain leading to fatigue and mild depression, leading to more tension and pain.

DO NOT SELF-TREAT FOR DEPRESSION

When we use the word "depression" in this chapter, we use it to describe the chronic fatigue and frustration that many people experience when going through a difficult, chronic, painful problem. This type of pain wears you down and can lead to a mild form of depression. This depression can lead to three problems:

▶ It makes it more difficult to bear the constant pain.
▶ It can increase inflammation in the body, which can lead to more pain.
▶ It can increase tension, which is often experienced as increased tightness in the neck and shoulder muscles.

The signs and symptoms of true medical depression include:

▶ Feeling sad and/or helpless
▶ Appetite or weight changes
▶ Significant sleep changes: either insomnia or sleeping too much
▶ Chronic fatigue or loss of energy
▶ Irritability
▶ Thoughts of hurting yourself or others
▶ Feelings of hopelessness
▶ Loss of interest in normal activities
▶ Loss of interest in sex

Talk to your doctor if you experience any of the problems listed in the accompanying box. In some rare instances, neck pain can be the presenting symptom of a true underlying depression or other psychiatric disorder. If you are suffering from depression or another psychiatric problem, or you are concerned that you might be, addressing it will make you feel much better, *and* it will also greatly help your neck pain. If you think you might fit into this category, you owe it to yourself and everyone around you to talk to your doctor.

You should not take SAM-e if you are taking any antidepressant medication, have bipolar disorder, have or are at risk for heart disease, are pregnant or thinking of becoming pregnant, nursing, or under the age of 18. One potential side effect of SAM-e is that it can raise the levels of *homocysteine* in the body, which has been associated with an increased risk of cardiovascular disease.

MONITORING SUPPLEMENT USAGE

It is a good idea to ask your doctor to monitor your blood chemistry with periodic renal and liver function tests whenever you are taking any supplement. Homocysteine is a chemical compound that is made from naturally occurring amino acids in the body. When taking SAM-e, it is a good idea to ask your doctor to periodically check your homocysteine level. If it is elevated, one way to lower it is with supplemental folate.

The other major drawback of SAM-e is the cost. The recommended dose is 800 mg once a day, which can cost more than $120 a month.

SHOULD YOU TAKE SAM-E FOR NECK PAIN?

You might benefit from taking SAM-e for your neck pain if:

► Cost is not an issue.

► You do not meet any of the contraindications listed in the accompanying box.

► You have had neck pain for more than 3 months.

If you meet these criteria, we suggest that you consider taking SAM-e for 3 months, in addition to following our recommendations for postural re-education, workstation adjustment, and exercise. If you are feeling better after 3 months, consider stopping SAM-e. If the pain returns, go back to taking the supplement. If the pain does not return, there is no need to take SAM-e again. As with glucosamine and chondroitin sulfate, the medical literature neither supports nor refutes the use of SAM-e for the treatment of chronic neck pain. Taking glucosamine and chondroitin sulfate is not a contraindication to taking SAM-e, because these three supplements can be taken together.

12

Acupuncture and Manual Manipulation

ACUPUNCTURE

If pure staying power were the measure of a good therapeutic approach, acupuncture would be a clear heavyweight champion treatment for most ailments. For thousands of years, acupuncture has been used for everything that ails and debilitates the human condition. However, staying power is not the only criterion used to measure the efficacy of a treatment. What is acupuncture, and how effective is it for neck pain?

There are many schools of acupuncture, each with its own specific traditions. It usually involves the placement of small needles into "acupuncture points" around the body in an effort to restore health. According to traditional Chinese medicine (TCM), the body consists of channels of energy, called *chi*. Disease results from a disruption in the flow of chi through these channels.

Acupuncture needles are used to access and manipulate the energy channels to restore the optimal flow of chi throughout the body. This is why an acupuncturist might place needles in your arms, legs, trunk, feet, ear, and scalp to treat your neck pain. From a TCM perspective, the pain is not necessarily "in your neck," but is a

According to traditional Chinese medicine (TCM), the body consists of channels of energy, called chi. Disease results from a disruption in the flow of chi through these channels.

result of blocked or excess energy that is manifested as neck pain. Restoring the flow is therefore more important than addressing the neck directly.

Modern Western science has had to grapple with both the staying power of acupuncture as a cure for many ailments and its apparent efficacy, especially for pain. In addition to the overwhelming volume of anecdotal reports of acupuncture being effective, recent research has supported its use for a variety of medical problems. In 1997, the National Institutes of Health (NIH) issued a consensus statement concluding that acupuncture was indicated for use in postoperative and chemotherapy-induced nausea and vomiting, as well as for dental pain, and that there was some evidence for its use in a variety of other pain conditions. The NIH also expressed the need and indication for further research, and several well-performed studies have demonstrated the efficacy of acupuncture for a variety of ailments.

Western scientists are left with this question: *If* acupuncture works, *why* does it work? They have been unable to dissect, palpate, image, or otherwise clearly identify the energy channels (meridians) that TCM practitioners believe exist. Some evidence has shown that certain major traditional acupuncture points possess some interesting properties. For example, one acupuncture point in the hand (in the web space between the thumb and pointer finger) contains an unusually large number of sympathetic fibers. One explanation for the effects of acupuncture is that the introduction of needles into the body stimulates it to produce increased endogenous endorphins, which stimulate the same receptors as *opioids*. Opioids are chemicals that the body naturally produces in order to decrease pain. This could help explain why localized acupuncture treatments for neck pain—meaning placing at least some of the needles directly into the neck—seem to reduce tension and pain in the neck and shoulders. However, the localized effects of opioids alone cannot explain all of the effects sometimes observed with acupuncture.

Regardless of the mechanism of action, the question remains, "Will acupuncture help my neck pain?"

Two recent studies on the use of acupuncture for chronic neck pain have suggested that it might. Further research is needed to offer an evidence-based recommendation as to whether acupuncture is clinically efficacious in the treatment of chronic neck pain. However, it can be said that the risks are minimal when acupuncture is performed by an experienced, expert practitioner.

Our recommendations regarding acupuncture are:

▶ *Never* use acupuncture to treat an ailment before getting a medical opinion first. Acupuncture is most dangerous when it is used *instead* of conventional medical care, rather than combined with it. The last thing you want is to control symptoms with acupuncture that might indicate a serious underlying medical condition. Take the time to get a medical doctor's opinion first.

▶ If you decide to have acupuncture treatments, a physician who is trained and certified in acupuncture should perform the treatments. (One of the authors is a medical doctor, and he is also trained in acupuncture.)

▶ Understand that acupuncture does not address the postural and biomechanical issues that might be contributing to your neck pain. Do not use acupuncture *instead* of postural re-education and exercises. In our experience, acupuncture is not a "quick fix." However, we also believe that it can be very helpful for some people. Acupuncture helps to relax the body and break up tight muscle spasms in the neck and shoulders—and it might just balance your energy.

▶ If you are interested in acupuncture, get a referral from your physician to a certified, experienced acupuncturist who is used to treating neck pain.

If you follow these recommendations, the major downside might be financial. Although some insurance companies cover acupuncture treatments, most do not. Also, any time a needle is inserted into the body, a potential risk exists for infection, bleeding, and/or increased pain. Needles placed in or around the lung can result in a collapsed lung, which is yet another important reason to see an experienced, certified professional.

MANUAL MANIPULATION

Several different forms of manipulation are available for neck pain, as well as different practitioners who are capable of performing them.

Chiropractors, doctors of osteopathic medicine, and medical doctors with special training are all trained to perform manipulations. The idea of manual manipulation is twofold: First, specific techniques relax the muscles, ligaments, and tendons. Second, they restore alignment in the spine. Manual manipulation can be very helpful for neck pain when used in conjunction with improved posture, improved overall biomechanics, and exercise. A few important cautions are worth noting, however.

Manual manipulation can be very helpful for neck pain when used in conjunction with improved posture, improved overall biomechanics, and exercise.

First, it is imperative that X-rays be taken before any manual manipulation of the neck is performed. If you have symptoms radiating into your arms, you should first have an MRI. In general, we do not recommend *high-velocity manipulations*, because they involve rapid, forceful, high-velocity movements of the cervical spine, which can cause serious injury. When a high-velocity manipulation to any body part is done, it should *only* be performed by someone who is well-trained, well-qualified, and very experienced.

It is important to realize that everyone has some "misalignment." If we examined 100 randomly selected people who have no pain, a significant number of them would have something "out of place" in their spines—either on physical examination or MRI. On average, about 40 of 100 people with no symptoms actually have herniated discs in their lower

A Caveat Regarding Manual Manipulation

Occasionally, a misalignment is so significant that—even in the absence of clinical symptoms—it needs to be treated. However, such treatment requires surgery rather than manual manipulation. This is extremely rare, and it is the exception rather than the rule.

back. The point is that simply being "out of alignment" is not something that requires treatment. The key is for a physician to be able to correlate misalignment with clinical symptoms and to treat appropriately.

For most people, the most important aspect of manipulation for neck pain is to relax the muscles, ligaments, and tendons—rather than realign them. Relaxing the muscles, combined with improved biomechanics and exercise, is very effective. When the muscles are strong but relaxed, and daily biomechanics are optimal, alignment tends to take care of itself—and so does pain.

13

Meditation

Imagine you are sitting by the beach with a drink in one hand and a good book in the other, the waves lapping gently around your ankles—the sun is warm, but the ocean breeze keeps you from getting hot. You sigh, because you know you have to get up soon and go to the pool-bar, where you'll order an afternoon snack. A dip in the pool and then you'll come back to the beach for a well-deserved nap. Neck pain? Oh, right—you used to have neck pain.

What is meditation—and can it really help your neck pain? In this chapter, we'll discuss one of the most powerful ways to heal yourself, and maybe even reach new heights of personal potential. Most people think of meditation as a state of supreme relaxation. In some respects, that's true. But in other ways, it couldn't be more false.

MEDITATION

Eckhart Tolle is a spiritual leader who has made Eastern philosophy much more accessible for millions of Westerners. He teaches us to think of the mind as a *tool*, just like the neck, arms, and legs are tools. You use your arms to carry things, your legs to walk, and your mind to think. Your mind instructs your arms to carry, to drive, to figure out how to get a promotion at work, and how to set up your new DVD player. If you are not your mind, then who are you? *You* are a spiritual entity. *You* inhabit a body that came complete with lots of tools, including a mind, legs, arms, and a heart.

Tolle teaches that you should make it a practice to divorce yourself from your mind and learn to watch and listen to your thoughts. *This is very similar to meditation,* and it is a hallmark of many Eastern philosophies.

Meditation is a profoundly relaxing state. However, to get to that state of relaxation, you need to make yourself hyperaware. Meditation lives only in the present. When meditating, you are aware of how you are feeling *now*. You are aware of the thoughts in your head, the breath moving in and out of your lungs, the sounds around you, the smells in the air, and the beating of your heart. You are *not* thinking about where you are going to go later tonight—or why your boss didn't appreciate the work you did on "Project X."

> Meditation is a profoundly relaxing state.

Meditation also affords you an excellent way to combat pain. In addition to becoming relaxed, you have the chance—indeed the obligation—to "watch your pain." This is a technique incorporated by the controversial best-selling author Dr. John Sarno at New York University, who uses this approach to treat people with a wide variety of musculoskeletal problems. When you are meditating, you are fully aware of all that is going on in the moment. When a thought comes into your head ("I forgot to buy milk"), you don't engage the thought ("Shoot—I have to go buy milk later today"). Instead, you watch the thought and let it pass as if it flashed on a screen and then went away. Similarly, when you have pain in your neck, watch the pain and place a label on it ("Pain"), and then try to get more specific. The pain is just left of midline. It is sharp—now dull—now burning—now gone. As you observe your pain, you will find that it has a way of moving slightly, subtly changing character—and sometimes even leaving. It is as if the pain is a dark shadow, and that by focusing the intense light beam of your consciousness on it and describing it in minute detail, you expose the shadow so that it goes away. Try it!

How Do You Meditate?

Start with a dark, quiet room and a comfortable chair—preferably one with a headrest. Set aside 15 minutes. Turn off your television, radio, cell phone, PDA, home phone, pager, and anything else that beeps, buzzes, or plays music. Take a slow breath in. Feel the breath entering your throat and descending into your lungs. Feel your chest expand and slowly contract. Focus on your breathing. When thoughts of the day's events enter your mind (and they inevitably will at first), let them pass. Return to your breathing. Focus. If your neck is hurting, *watch your pain.* Don't give in to it. Don't attach an emotion to it. Just watch it, and observe that it hurts. Where? What is the character of it? Don't start thinking about how long it has hurt or what made it worse during the day. Just focus on how it feels *right now.*

Meditating is extremely simple, as you can see. But it is also very hard! Watching your thoughts and focusing on your breathing is not as easy as it sounds. Please don't lose confidence. If you keep at it, once a day, you'll get it.

Typically, our patients report feeling better and more relaxed after doing this for 1–2 weeks. The relaxation begins during the meditation and often lasts for a few hours afterward. However, as the person gets back into the world, the tension often mounts again, and the pain and angst return. After 3–6 weeks, the relaxation and pain relief should start to last for longer—sometimes several hours. It takes a few months for most people to become avid medita-tors. But once you start to "get it," meditation can become addicting.

Disentangling yourself from your thoughts can be a great unburdening.

There is no downside to trying this except for the time it takes. One of the upsides is that most people realize—often for the first time—just how wrapped up in their head they really are. Disentangling yourself from your thoughts can be a great unburdening.

Once you become adept at "watching your thoughts" and being able to disengage almost at will from your emotions, you will be able to use the technique throughout the day. Instead of carrying stress and tension in your shoulders, like all of your colleagues, you'll be able to exhale and let it go. Each night or morning (or both) when you meditate, you'll re-energize yourself and your spirit.

A meditation or relaxation tape can be very helpful as you begin your meditation journey.

14

Concluding Thoughts—Putting It All Together

HOPE AND HELP

Neck pain is a serious national health problem, with serious consequences. It can be disabling; it can cause difficulty for loved ones and
co-workers; and it can be depressing. Many people with chronic neck
pain tell us that even their personalities have changed for the worse over
time because of neck pain—they tell us they no longer feel like the person they once were. Many of them are barely into their 30s!

We believe that many of these people suffer needlessly and that
there is hope for all of them. Many times the solution is relatively simple, as in Ted's case. Other times, things can be more complicated, as for
Sonia. No matter how difficult, we believe there is hope and help for
anyone with neck pain.

But first you have to recognize that you just can't do it alone.
Much of the advice we give regarding breaking bad habits and institut-
ing neck support programs might seem like common sense. But it really
isn't. Many of our patients are brilliant and successful people but—for
whatever reason—they cannot solve the problem of their poor necks
alone. If neck pain keeps you from doing the things you love—from
being the *real* person you are—try following the recommendations in
Chapter 3. If you have any of the "red flag symptoms" or your pain per-

sists, call your doctor for a full and complete evaluation. On occasion, it might take a few follow-up evaluations and some trial and error before the doctor can really pin down a diagnosis. But stick with it. Neck pain is very responsive to treatment most of the time, but only after an accurate diagnosis is made.

As we conclude, we must return to our first principle one last time: Respect your neck. Remember, it gives you everything it has to give. Its capabilities are astounding, but it also demands much of *you*. When we take it for granted, we pay the price—many of us every day. But this does not have to be the case. You *will* see positive results if you make good neck hygiene as much a part of your life as brushing your teeth.

We hope that reading this book has given you a new appreciation for your neck and all it can do—and can't do. Awareness is your best defense. E-mail, computers, and cell phones are not going anywhere anytime soon, and we have to adapt to our environment. This has always been true. But you *can* and *will* overcome the neck pain epidemic! You have already made a good start by reading this book.

We wish you the best of health, because with good health all things are possible.

Index

Note: Boldface numbers indicate illustrations.

acetaminophen (Tylenol), 4, 63, 89–90
acetylsalicylic acid (aspirin), 88
acupuncture, 113–116
Advil. *See* ibuprofen
aerobic exercise, 47, 56
Aleve. *See* Naprosyn
analgesics, 88, 89–90
anatomy of the neck, 13–14
   bones/vertebrae of cervical spine in,
     17–21, **17**, **19**, **66**, **94**
   coordination of movement and,
     16–21
   epidural space in, 97–98
   facet joints in, 18, 27–28
   foramen of vertebrae in, 18
   intervertebral discs in, 18
   ligaments and tendons in, 18,
     26–27
   misalignments in, manipulation
     and, 116–117
   movement capability and, 14–16, **15**
   muscles in, 14–16, **14**, **15**, 23–26
   nerves and, 18–21, **19**, **20**
   spinal cord and, 18–21
anesthetics, topical (Lidoderm
    patches), 88
arm press exercise, 53, **53**
arthritis, 106
aspirin, 4, 88
atlantoaxial joint, 60

back strengthening/stretching exercise,
    47–49, **48**

Ben-Gay, 88
Bextra, 89
bicycling precautions, 56
blood tests, 62
bones/vertebrae of cervical spine,
    17–21, **17**, **19**, **66**, **94**
Botox. *See* botulinum toxin (Botox,
    Myobloc) injections
botulinum toxin (Botox, Myobloc)
    injections, 84–85
bowel/bladder function changes, 99
breathing and exercise, 46–47

cancer, 60
Capzasin-P, 88
cartilage, 106
Celebrex, 89
cervical collars, 73–75, **74**
cervical discography, 99
cervical spine bones, 17–21, **17**, **19**, **66**,
    94
chi and acupuncture, 113
chin tuck exercise, 53
chiropractic, 116–117
clavicle, 15
coccyx, 18
collars, 73–75, **74**
computed tomography. *See* CT scans
computer use and neck pain, vii, 5–6,
    9–12, **9**, 24, **26**, 38–42, **39**, **40**, **41**
Cooper, Grant, 106
coordination of neck movements,
    16–21

COX-2 inhibitors, 89
CT scans, 99

depression, 109
desk height, 38–42, **39, 40, 41**
diagnosing causes of neck pain,
    123–124
diclofenac (Voltaren), 88
diclofenac epolamine patch (Flector),
    88
discs. *See* intervertebral discs
doctor's visit, 59–70
    patient history (sample) in, 62–68
    physical exam during, 65–66
    questions the doctor may ask dur-
        ing, 61–62
    red flag signs and symptoms war-
        ranting, 60–61, 82–83, 123
    risk–benefit analysis of treatment
        during, 68–70
    second opinions and, 98–99, **98**
    symptoms requiring a, 59–60, 123
    symptoms review during, 64–65,
        123
dorsal ramus nerves, 95

epidemic of neck pain, 3–12
epidural space, 97–98
epidural steroid injections, 81,
    97–98
ergonomics at work, 38–42, **39, 40, 41**
evolution and the neck, 6–7, 21–22
exercise, 21–22, 45–57, 68–70, 100.
    See also posture
    10-minute program for the neck,
        47–57
    aerobic, stretching, and strengthen-
        ing components of, 47, 56
    arm presses, 53, **53**
    back strengthening/stretching,
        47–49, **48**
    bicycling as, 56
    breathing in, 46–47
    chin tuck, 53
    doctor's ok for, 45
    forward neck stretch, 51, **51**
    forward neck stretch, standing, 52,
        52

general principles of, 46–47
    pain and, 47
    physical therapy and, 72–73
    sideways neck stretch, 49, **50**
    TheraBand used in, 45–46, **46**, 54,
        54
    wall presses, 55–57, **55**

facet joints, 18, 27–28, **28**, 94–96
    dorsal ramus nerves and, 95
    injections into, 95–96
    medial branch block in, 95–96
    pain in, 27–28, 94–96
    radiofrequency neurotomy and, 96,
        97
FDA approval of treatments, 85
fevers/chills, 60
Flector. *See* diclofenac epolamine
    patch
foramen of vertebrae, 18
forward neck stretch, 51, **51**
forward neck stretch, standing, 52, **52**

glucosamine and chondroitin
    sulfate, 105–108

high-intensity zones, 99
homocysteine levels and SAM-e, 110
hope for neck pain, 123–124

ibuprofen (Advil, Motrin), 4, 63, 88
Icy Hot, 88
imaging studies, 62, 80–83. *See also*
    CT scans, MRIs, X-rays
impact of neck pain on lifestyle, 4,
    7–8
Indocin. *See* indomethacin
indomethacin (Indocin), 88
infections, 62
injections into neck/spine, 81, 83–85,
    86, 93–101
    facet joint, 95–96
    medial branch block as, 83, 95–96
    radiofrequency neurotomy and, 96
    steroid injections, 97–98
    trigger points and, 83–84, 86, 100
insertion of muscle, 15
intervertebral discs, 18

lidocaine (Lidoderm), 88
lidocaine injections, 84
Lidoderm. *See* lidocaine
ligaments of the neck, 18, 26–27

magnetic resonance imaging. *See* MRIs
manipulation, 116–117
manual manipulation, 116–117
massage, 116–117
mastoid process, 16
mattress selection, 42–43
medial branch block, 83, 95–96
medication, 69–70, 87–91
  analgesic, 89–90
  muscle relaxant, 90–91
  narcotic type, 90
  oral, 88–89
  side effects of, 88–89
  systemic absorption of, 87
  topical, 87–88
  "window of opportunity" provided
    by, 91
meditation, 119–122
misalignments of spine, 116–117
Motrin. *See* ibuprofen
movement capability of the neck,
    14–16, **15**
MRIs, 62, 80–83, 94, 99
muscle relaxants, 88, 90–91
muscles of the neck, 14–16, **14, 15,**
    23–26
muscular neck pain, 23–26
Myobloc. *See* botulinum toxin (Botox,
    Myobloc) injections

Naprosyn (Aleve), 88
narcotic pain killers, 90
National Institutes of Health (NIH)
    on acupuncture, 114
nerves of the neck, 18–21, **19, 20**
neurologic deficit, 70, 82–83
night sweats, 60
nonsteroidal anti-inflammatory drugs
    (NSAIDs), 69–70, 88, 89
NSAIDs. *See* nonsteroidal anti-inflam-
    matory drugs
numbness/tingling sensations, 59,
    82–83, 99

off-label use of Botox in neck pain, 85
oral medications, 88–89
origin of muscle, 15
over-the-counter medications, 69–70,
    88. *See also* analgesics

pain during exercise, 47
pain medication, 4. *See also* medication
painkillers. *See* analgesics
patient history in diagnosis, 62–68
pectoral muscles, 24
percutaneous procedures, 97
physical examination, 65–66
physical therapy, 72–73
pillow selection, 42–43
posture, 8–12, **9,** 24–26, **25, 26,** 31–43,
    82, 100. *See also* exercise
  holding or maintaining, 42
  sitting, **32,** 35–38, **37, 38**
  sleeping and, 42–43
  standing, 32–33, **33, 34**
  walking, 33–35, **35, 36**
  workstation setup for improving,
    38–42, **39, 40, 41**
prednisone, 89
prevalence of neck pain, 3–12

questions the doctor may ask you,
    61–62

radiating pain down arm, 59
radiofrequency neurotomy, 96, 97
rashes and neck pain, 60
red flag signs and symptoms, 60–61,
    82–83, 123
rheumatoid arthritis, 60
rhomboid muscles, 24
risk–benefit analysis of treatment,
    68–70

S-adenosylmethionine (SAM-e),
    108–111
SAM-e. *See* S-adenosylmethionine
    (SAM-e)
Sarno, John, 120
second opinions, 98–99
sedentary lifestyle and neck pain, vii,
    6–12, 21–22. *See also* exercise

sideways neck stretch, 49, **50**
sitting posture, 24–26, **25, 26,** 32,
    35–38, **37, 38**
sleep
    cervical collar use during, 75
    good posture and, 42–43
    interrupted by pain, 60
spinal cord, 18–21
standing posture, 32–33, **33, 34**
sternocleidomastoid muscles, 15–16,
    15
sternum, 15
steroid injections, 81, 84, 97–98
steroids, 89
strengthening exercises, 47
stretching exercises, 47
supplements, 105–111
    glucosamine and chondroitin
        sulfate, 105–108
    S-adenosylmethionine (SAM-e),
        108–111
surgery, 81–82, 98
    second opinion essential in, 98–99
symptoms requiring a doctor's visit,
    59–70, 99, 123
symptoms review by doctor, 64–65
systemic absorption of medications, 87

telephone use and neck pain, vii, 5–6,
    9–12
Ten-Minute Exercise Program, 47–57,
    48
tendons in the neck, 18, 26–27
TheraBand exerciser, 45–46, **46,** 54, **54**

topical medications, 87
traditional Chinese medicine (TCM)
    and acupuncture, 113–116
tramadol (Ultram), 90
transverse ligament, 60
trapezius muscles, 24
trigger points, 62, 83–84, 86, 100
Tylenol. *See* acetaminophen

Ultram. *See* tramadol
unstable neck injuries, 75

vertebrae, 17–21, **17, 19, 66, 94**
Vioxx, 89
Voltaren. *See* diclofenac

walking posture, 33–35, **35, 36**
wall press exercises, 55–57, **55**
weakness in arms/neck, 59, 82–83, 99
weight loss/gain, 60
whiplash injury, 27
"window of opportunity" provided by
    medications, 91
workplace environment and neck
    pain, vii, 5–12, 31–43, 82. *See also*
    posture, exercise
    ergonomics and, 38–42, **39, 40, 41**
    workstation setup for improving
        posture, 38–42, **39, 40, 41**
worsening pain, 60

X-rays, 62, 99
    injections guided by. *See* injections
    normal cervical spine, 66

NOTES

Notes